Workbook for use with
# Medical Coding Fundamentals

# Workbook for use with
# Medical Coding Fundamentals

**Susan Goldsmith, CPC, CPC-H, CPC-P, CPC-I, CCP, CCS-P, CPEHR**

**Marc Leib, MD, JD**

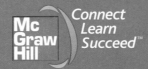

Mc Graw Hill

*Connect
Learn
Succeed*™

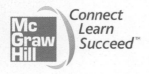

WORKBOOK FOR USE WITH MEDICAL CODING FUNDAMENTALS, FIRST EDITION
SUSAN GOLDSMITH AND MARC LEIB

1 2 3 4 5 6 7 8 9 0 QDB/QDB 1 0 9 8 7 6 5 4 3 2

ISBN       978-0-07-740117-7
MHID       0-07-740117-4

All brand or product names are trademarks or registered trademarks of their respective companies.

The Internet addresses listed in the text were accurate at the time of publication. The inclusion of a website does not indicate an endorsement by the authors or McGraw-Hill, and McGraw-Hill does not guarantee the accuracy of the information presented at these sites.

CPT five-digit codes, nomenclature, and other data are copyright © 2011, American Medical Association. All rights reserved. No fee schedules, basic unit, relative values, or related listings are included in CPT. The AMA assumes no liability for the data contained herein.

CPT codes are based on CPT 2012.
HCPCS codes are based on HCPCS 2012.
ICD-9-CM codes are based on ICD-9-CM 2012.

www.mhhe.com

# TABLE OF CONTENTS

*Preface*  vi

**1**  Medical Terminology, Anatomy, and Physiology  1

## PART I:  ICD-9-CM and ICD-10-CM

**2**  Introduction to ICD-9-CM  14
**3**  ICD-9-CM Chapter-Specific Guidelines, Part I: Chapters 1–10  20
**4**  ICD-9-CM Chapter-Specific Guidelines, Part II: Chapters 11–19  29
**5**  Introduction to ICD-10-CM and ICD-10-PCS  36

## PART II:  CPT and HCPCS

**6**  Introduction to CPT  42
**7**  Modifiers  53
**8**  Evaluation and Management Services, Part I: Structure and Guidance  61
**9**  Evaluation and Management Services, Part II: Code Selection  68
**10**  Anesthesia Services  76
**11**  Radiology Services  84
**12**  Surgery Codes: Coding for Surgical Procedures on Specific Organ Systems
    Module 12.1 General and Integumentary System  93
    Module 12.2 Musculoskeletal System  99
    Module 12.3 Respiratory, Cardiovascular, Hemic, and Lymphatic Systems; Mediastinum and Diaphragm  105
    Module 12.4 Digestive System  112
    Module 12.5 Urinary System, Male and Female Genital Systems, and Maternity Care and Delivery  118
    Module 12.6 Endocrine, Nervous, Ocular, and Auditory Systems  125
**13**  Pathology and Laboratory Services  132
**14**  Medicine Services  140
**15**  Introduction to the Healthcare Common Procedure Coding System (HCPCS)  148

## PART III:  Practicum

**16**  Putting It All Together  155

# PREFACE

The *Workbook for use with Medical Coding Fundamentals* is intended to strengthen, reinforce, and expand student learning of the skills and concepts presented in the text, *Medical Coding Fundamentals*. The workbook complements and follows the same learning outcomes as the text.

The Key Terms activities help strengthen students' vocabulary for each chapter. Exam Review questions provide additional hands-on practice with the coding concepts presented in each chapter while familiarizing students with the format of certification exams. Applying Your Skills exercises and Case Studies build coding ability and analytical skills as students learn to identify the codes in each scenario. Thinking It Through questions ask students to go beyond code selection and think critically about aspects of coding.

Instructors may choose to use sections of the workbook in class, for example, using the Key Terms section as a pretest. Instructors may select individual assignments for each chapter, depending on the progress of the class, or assign specific activities to students who might be having difficulty grasping certain themes. For example, the instructor might assign all students the Applying Your Skills exercises to reinforce the reading of each chapter, or the Exam Review questions could be used by students individually or as a class as a pretest before chapter or part tests. The additional activities could be used in their entirety, or portions may be selected to highlight individual concepts from the text.

The Instructor Manual for *Medical Coding Fundamentals* provides keys to all activities. Instructors can access the Instructor Manual via the book's Online Learning Center (OLC) website, **www.mhhe.com/goldsmith**.

## Organization of the Workbook

*Medical Coding Fundamentals* consists of a review chapter followed by three parts. The *Workbook for use with Medical Coding Fundamentals* is organized in the same way.

| Part | Coverage |
| --- | --- |
| **Medical Terminology, Anatomy, and Physiology** | Chapter 1 provides an overview of anatomical systems, basic physiology, and medical terminology, including common prefixes and suffixes. |
| **One: ICD-9-CM and ICD-10-CM** | Chapters 2 to 5 cover the format and guidelines of the ICD-9-CM code set. The student is walked through the use of ICD-9-CM to assign diagnosis codes. The material introduces the transition to ICD-10-CM and ICD-10-PCS, along with basic information about code assignment in the new code set. |
| **Two: CPT and HCPCS** | Chapters 6 to 15 describe the format and guidelines of the CPT and HCPCS code sets. These chapters explain the process for selecting modifiers and E/M codes. The material includes comprehensive, modular coverage of surgical procedures as they relate to body systems. |
| **Three: Practicum** | Chapter 16 offers additional, concentrated coding practice. |

# CodeitRightOnline™: Your Online Coding Tool

So that your students can gain experience with the use of an online coding tool, they will have access for a 29-day period to CodeitRightOnline, produced by Contexo Media, a division of Access Intelligence.

## Features

The general features offered with a subscription include the following:

- *CodeitRightOnline Search.* The ability to find a CPT, HCPCS Level II, and ICD-9-CM code either using the index or tabular search sections, by code terminology, description, keyword, or code number. Additionally, the Single Search feature allows you to locate all codes related to a particular term.
- *Fully Customizable.* Provides note capability, local coverage determination (LCD) customization, personalized searches and fee schedules, and specialty-specific code sets.
- *Coding Crosswalks.* Essential coding links from CPT codes to ICD-9-CM to HCPCS Level II codes and to anesthesia codes.
- *Articles.* Articles from CMS, OIG, carriers, intermediaries, payers, and other government websites along with newsletter articles from AMA, AHA, Decision Health, Coding Institute, and others.
- LCD/NCD codes for a local state carrier; Medicare's payment policy indicators; and, of course, CPT, HCPCS Level II, and ICD-9-CM codes with full descriptions and plain English definitions.
- *ICD-10-CM/PCS Code Sets.* Help you prepare for 2013 mandatory implementation with ICD-10-CM/PCS full code sets and descriptions.
- *NCCI Edits Validator™.* Validates codes to help you remain in compliance with the correct coding guidelines established by the Centers for Medicare and Medicaid Services (CMS).
- *Automatic Updates.* Ensures that CodeitRightOnline contains the most up-to-date, real-time information.
- *Build-A-Code™.* Allows students to build codes from the ground up, helping them understand how ICD-10 codes are constructed.
- *Click-A-Dex™.* Helps index searches for easy future reference.
- *Comprehensive Medicare Resource.* Contains LCD and national coverage determination (NCD) information, contact information for a comprehensive list of Medicare providers, and information on how to bill for procedures allowed by Medicare's Physician Quality Reporting Initiative (PQRI) program.
- *ABC Codes and Descriptions.* Provide access to the alternative medicine codes you need to describe services, remedies, and/or supplies required during patient visits.
- *Educational Games and Learning Tools.* Help reinforce the student's knowledge of anatomy.

McGraw Hill connect plus+
Enhance your learning by completing these exercises
and more at mcgrawhillconnect.com!

PREFACE        vii

## Using the Online Coding Tool

Go to **www.codeitrightonline.com** to complete the steps needed to begin. The following screen will appear.

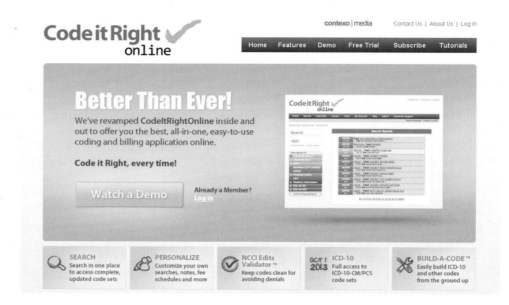

Click the *Free Trial* tab at the top right-hand corner of the screen. On the page that appears, enter your name, e-mail address, school, phone, and address. Next, click *Use account contact information* for your account administrator information, a one-time process that optimizes CodeitRightOnline for your particular location. Choose a user name and password you will remember. Next, read the terms and conditions, including the AMA agreement. After accepting the terms and conditions, click *Continue*. You will then receive an e-mail containing an activation link. Clicking the link activates your account. From that page, click the *Click here* link to sign in with the account information you selected. This will take you to the CodeitRightOnline home page—you're in!

These actions set up your trial subscription. Now, to use the online coding tool to locate codes, click *Search* and select the appropriate code set. Next, choose the start point for your code search. For example, select *ICD-9-CM Vol 1, 2 and Vol 3* in the Show Results For box, and enter the term *Fracture,* and click *Search.* CodeitRightOnline will return a list of the various fracture entries for your selection. To see how it works, choose *Fracture of Ribs, Closed,* and click the code number to review the tabular list entry.

# ACKNOWLEDGMENTS

Thanks to the instructors and reviewers who have provided feedback on the workbook's first edition. Special thanks are due to Mary Cantwell, Deborah Kenney, JanMarie Malik, Selinda McCumbers, Edward O'Beirne, and Angela Suarez for their work on the exercises.

A full list of reviewers can be found in the acknowledgments section of the main text, *Medical Coding Fundamentals*.

# TO THE STUDENT

The workbook is designed to help you prepare for your career as a medical coder, an integral role in providing quality healthcare to patients. The workbook, which accompanies your *Medical Coding Fundamentals* text, is intended to help you strengthen, reinforce, and expand your learning of the skills and concepts presented in the text.

To improve or expand your medical vocabulary, focus on the Key Terms exercises, which can also be used as a pretest. Other workbook activities focus on applying what you have learned in the text and/or class. Thinking It Through consists of critical-thinking questions to help you assess what you have mastered and what you still need to study. Exam Review questions give you extra coding practice and help you prepare for coding certification exams.

Welcome to the world of healthcare!

# MEDICAL TERMINOLOGY, ANATOMY, AND PHYSIOLOGY

## Learning Outcomes

*After completing this chapter, students should be able to:*

**1.1** Differentiate word elements, including word roots, prefixes, and suffixes, and understand how these elements are used to construct complex medical terms.

**1.2** Recognize and define commonly used eponyms, abbreviations, and acronyms.

**1.3** Identify anatomical structures and the systems to which they belong.

**1.4** Describe how the adoption of ICD-10-CM in 2013 will affect the use of medical terminology.

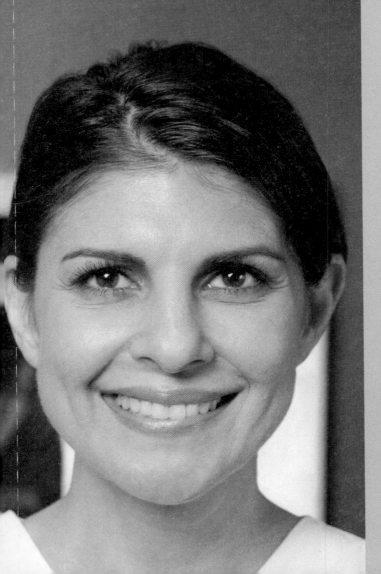

## Introduction

Before learning to report medical services, procedures, and supplies, it is necessary to understand medical terminology, anatomy, and physiology. You may already have had separate classes covering these subjects, or this might be your first introduction to these important topics.

Learning medical terminology is similar to learning a foreign language. The words are new and unfamiliar. The meaning of many of these terms must be learned and memorized. There are also rules for the medical terminology language, mostly involving how these words are constructed from root words, prefixes, and suffixes. Coders must be able to recognize individual word parts, break words down into their components, and construct medical terms from components.

*Anatomy* is the study of the physical structures of the body, including those that make up the musculoskeletal system, organs, and glands. The study of anatomy is usually divided into the study of specific systems, including the integumentary, musculoskeletal, cardiovascular, lymphatic, respiratory, digestive, urinary, reproductive, nervous, endocrine, and hemic systems. Physiology is the study of how these anatomical structures function in the living body.

# Key Terms

Define each of the following key terms in the space provided.

**1.** [LO 1.3]  Urinary system _____

_____

**2.** [LO 1.1]  Root word _____

_____

**3.** [LO 1.1]  Combining vowel _____

_____

**4.** [LO 1.3]  Organ _____

_____

**5.** [LO 1.4]  Diagnosis code _____

_____

**6.** [LO 1.3]  Heart _____

_____

**7.** [LO 1.2]  Eponym _____

_____

**8.** [LO 1.3]  Deoxygenated _____

_____

**9.** [LO 1.4]  ICD-9-CM _____

_____

**10.** [LO 1.3]  Anatomy _____

_____

**11.** [LO 1.3]  Physiology _____

_____

**12.** [LO 1.1]  Combining form _____

_____

**13.** [LO 1.3]  Glands _____

_____

**14.** [LO 1.3]  Frontal plane _____

_____

**15.** [LO 1.3]  Sagittal plane _____

_____

**16.** [LO 1.3]  Transverse plane _____

_____

**17.** [LO 1.3]  Integumentary system _____

_____

**18.** [LO 1.3]  Cardiovascular system _____

_____

**19.** [LO.1]  Suffix _____

_____

**20.** [LO 1.3]  Arterial system _____

_____

**21.** [LO 1.3]  Capillaries _____

_____

**22.** [LO 1.3]  Venous system _____

_____

**23.** [LO 1.3]  Oxygenated _____

_____

**24.** [LO 1.2]  Abbreviation _____

_____

**25.** [LO 1.3]  Lymphatic system _____

_____

**26.** [LO 1.3]  Respiratory system _____

_____

**27.** [LO 1.3]  Digestive system _____

_____

**28.** [LO 1.1]  Word elements _____

_____

**29.** [LO 1.3]  Reproductive system _____

_____

**30.** [LO 1.3]  Nervous system _____

_____

**31.** [LO 1.3]  Endocrine system _____

_____

**32.** [LO 1.3]  Hemic system _____

_____

**33.** [LO 1.2]  Acronym _____

_____

**34.** [LO 1.4]  ICD-10-CM _____

_____

**35.** [LO 1.1]  Prefix _____

_____

## Exam Review

Select the letter that best completes each statement or question.

1. [LO 1.1]  Which of the following is often used to facilitate pronunciation of a medical term that is comprised of several parts?
   a. Root word
   b. Combining vowel
   c. Prefix
   d. Suffix

**2.** [LO 1.1]  Which of the following may indicate location, position, time, or number within a medical term?

    **a.** Suffix
    **b.** Root word
    **c.** Prefix
    **d.** Eponym

**3.** [LO 1.1]  Which of the following usually indicates a procedure, condition, disorder, or disease?

    **a.** Root word
    **b.** Abbreviation
    **c.** Eponym
    **d.** Suffix

**4.** [LO 1.1]  Which of the following may change the way a word is used within a sentence?

    **a.** Root word
    **b.** Acronym
    **c.** Suffix
    **d.** Prefix

**5.** [LO 1.1]  Determining the meaning of a medical term involves which of the following?

    **a.** Reading the entire word
    **b.** Examining each separate word part
    **c.** Recombining the word elements
    **d.** Understanding it in context of a document only

**6.** [LO 1.1]  Which of the following was named for the physician who first described the condition?

    **a.** Lou Gehrig disease
    **b.** Parkinson disease
    **c.** Down syndrome
    **d.** Both *b* and *c*

**7.** [LO 1.1]  Which of the following describes an acronym?

    **a.** A shortened version of a word
    **b.** The first letters of each word in a multiple-word term
    **c.** A word typically written with capital letters
    **d.** Shorthand versions of words like *treatment* (Tx), *diagnosis* (Dx), and *prescription* (Rx)

**8.** [LO 1.1]  If *end-* means "within" and *arter-* means "artery," what does *-ectomy* mean in the word *endarterectomy*?

    **a.** Removal of arterial plaque
    **b.** Surgical incision
    **c.** Surgical excision
    **d.** Arterial constriction

**9.** [LO 1.1]  What is the meaning of *pneum, pneumo,* or *pneumon* within a medical term?

    **a.** Respiratory condition
    **b.** Breathing
    **c.** Air/lung
    **d.** Inflammation

**10.** [LO 1.1]  Which of the following correctly defines *nephrolithiasis* when breaking down the medical term into its component parts?

    **a.** Kidney stones
    **b.** Renal condition
    **c.** Removal of kidney
    **d.** Renal lithotripsy

**11.** [LO 1.1] Which of the following is a distinction between *intra-* and *inter-*?

    **a.** Surface and outside
    **b.** Between and inside
    **c.** Within and during
    **d.** Inside and between

**12.** [LO 1.1] A variety of endogenous substrates are normally produced by the body. These include thyroid hormone, estrogen, insulin, etc. However, a patient may not make enough of a particular substance and may therefore be required to take an exogenous form such as a prescribed hormone replacement or medication. Which of the following correctly distinguishes *endo-* from *exo-*?

    **a.** Outside and inside
    **b.** Inside and outside
    **c.** Beginning and end
    **d.** Natural and unnatural

**13.** [LO 1.1] Certain bacteria normally live in the gastrointestinal tract. They perform a number of necessary functions. Those bacteria are said to be endogenous and maintain a symbiotic relationship with us unless disturbed by immunosuppressive agents/disease. Ectopathogens such as parasites, fungi, or viruses may be acquired when there is an opportunity for infection. Which of the following is the distinguishing factor between *endo-* and *ecto-*?

    **a.** Inside and outside
    **b.** Outside and inside
    **c.** Beginning and end
    **d.** Natural and unnatural

**14.** [LO 1.3] Which of the following is important for medical coders to know as they interpret medical terms within the context of the medical record?

    **a.** The biochemical changes that occur in the body which lead to disease
    **b.** Names and locations of anatomical structures and their relation to each other
    **c.** The clinical implications of disease and care management for healthcare outcomes
    **d.** The patient's prognosis after being diagnosed with a disease

**15.** [LO 1.3] Which of the following must a coder understand in order to determine the correct diagnostic code assignment?

    **a.** The prevalence of disease as reported in a geographic area
    **b.** The services medically necessary for diagnostic code linkage
    **c.** Whether or not the diagnosis was present on admission
    **d.** The number of medications prescribed for each condition

**16.** [LO 1.1] The term *pneumo-* is a(n) _____.

    **a.** Suffix
    **b.** Prefix
    **c.** Combining form
    **d.** Anatomy

**17.** [LO 1.1] To which anatomical location does *crani-* refer?

    **a.** Brain
    **b.** Skull
    **c.** Kidney
    **d.** Gland

**18.** [LO 1.1] *Card/i* refers to which part of the body?

    **a.** Kidney
    **b.** Ovaries
    **c.** Testes
    **d.** Heart

**19.** [LO 1.1]  *Nephr/o-* is a prefix meaning _____.

    **a.** Lungs
    **b.** Kidney
    **c.** Gallbladder
    **d.** Liver

**20.** [LO 1.1]  What does the suffix *-megaly* mean?

    **a.** Inflammation
    **b.** Infection
    **c.** Enlargement
    **d.** Disease

**21.** [LO 1.1]  The prefix *orchi-* refers to which anatomical location?

    **a.** Ovaries
    **b.** Testes
    **c.** Brain
    **d.** Lungs

**22.** [LO 1.1]  If Melissa has hyperthyroidism, she has _____ thyroid hormone.

    **a.** Excessive
    **b.** Too little
    **c.** Normal
    **d.** Deficient

**23.** [LO 1.1]  The suffix *-ectomy* means _____.

    **a.** Incision
    **b.** Suture
    **c.** Removal
    **d.** Opening

**24.** [LO 1.1]  The suffix *-emesis* means _____.

    **a.** Nausea
    **b.** Pain
    **c.** Inflammation
    **d.** Vomiting

**25.** [LO 1.1]  *Brady-* is a prefix that means _____.

    **a.** Fast
    **b.** Slow
    **c.** Abnormal
    **d.** Rhythm

**26.** [LO 1.1]  The prefix *supra-* means _____.

    **a.** Below
    **b.** Distal
    **c.** Proximal
    **d.** Above

**27.** [LO 1.1]  *Retro-* is a prefix that means _____.

    **a.** Above
    **b.** Below
    **c.** Behind
    **d.** Forward

**28.** [LO 1.1]  *Intra-* in the term *intramuscular* means _____.

    **a.** Within
    **b.** Above

   **c.** Distal

   **d.** Under

**29.** [LO 1.1] *Pruritis* has the suffix *-itis*, which means _____.

   **a.** Swelling

   **b.** Inflammation

   **c.** Redness

   **d.** Bruising

**30.** [LO 1.1] *Arthro-* is a prefix that means _____.

   **a.** Arthritis

   **b.** Movement

   **c.** Ligament

   **d.** Joint

**31.** [LO 1.3] The term *dyspnea* refers to a disorder of the _____ system.

   **a.** Circulatory

   **b.** Pulmonary

   **c.** Lymphatic

   **d.** Digestive

**32.** [LO 1.3] Mr. Montblanc presents with pain in the joints. His physician diagnoses his condition as arthralgia. What body system is affected by this condition?

   **a.** Pulmonary

   **b.** Cardiac

   **c.** Musculoskeletal

   **d.** Renal

**33.** [LO 1.1] Mr. Montblanc also has an arthroscopic procedure performed on his knees. What does the suffix *-scope* mean?

   **a.** Excision

   **b.** To visualize

   **c.** Incision

   **d.** Operation

**34.** [LO 1.3] The combining term *-myo-* in cardiomyopathy refers to what body part?

   **a.** Cardiovascular

   **b.** Pulmonary

   **c.** Heart muscle

   **d.** Neurological

**35.** [LO 1.3] What body system is affected in a patient with a collection of clear fluid known as lymph?

   **a.** Lymphatic

   **b.** Neurological

   **c.** Pulmonary

   **d.** Integumentary

**36.** [LO 1.3] Elaine has asthma. This is a disorder of the _____.

   **a.** Cardiovascular system

   **b.** Reproductive system

   **c.** Integumentary system

   **d.** Pulmonary system

**37.** [LO 1.3] A patient is exhibiting tachypnea. This refers to which body system?

   **a.** Cardiovascular

   **b.** Respiratory

   **c.** Nephrotic

   **d.** Endocrine

**38.** [LO 1.3] The term *gastralgia* can be broken down and defined in which of the following ways?
   **a.** Liver/pain
   **b.** Stomach/pain
   **c.** Intestinal/pain
   **d.** Gallbladder/pain

**39.** [LO 1.2] To which body system does the term *hydronephrosis* refer?
   **a.** Renal system
   **b.** Nervous system
   **c.** Respiratory
   **d.** Gastrointestinal

**40.** [LO 1.1, 1.3] Mrs. Landis visits a physician, complaining of heartburn and chronic acid reflux. Her physician recommends an esophagogastroduodenoscopy. This procedure involves which body system?
   **a.** Nervous system
   **b.** Gastrointestinal system
   **c.** Cardiovascular system
   **d.** Reproductive system

## Identifying Word Parts

Identify each of the following word parts as prefix, suffix, or root word, and then define the term.

**1.** [LO 1.1] angi
   Prefix/suffix/root: _root_
   Definition: _Vessel_

**2.** [LO 1.1] brachi
   Prefix/suffix/root: _root_
   Definition: _arm_

**3.** [LO 1.1] chole
   Prefix/suffix/root: _root_
   Definition: _gallbladder_

**4.** [LO 1.1] cheil
   Prefix/suffix/root: _root_
   Definition: _lip_

**5.** [LO 1.1] diaphor
   Prefix/suffix/root: _root_
   Definition: _sweat_

**6.** [LO 1.1] laryng
   Prefix/suffix/root: _root_
   Definition: _larynx_

**7.** [LO 1.1] nephr
   Prefix/suffix/root: _root_
   Definition: _kidney_

**8.** [LO 1.1] rhino
   Prefix/suffix/root: _root_
   Definition: _nose_

**9.** [LO 1.1] vesico
   Prefix/suffix/root: _root_
   Definition: _bladder or sac_

**10.** [LO 1.1] olig
Prefix/suffix/root: _root_
Definition: _scanty or few_

**11.** [LO 1.1] ictal
Prefix/suffix/root: _____
Definition: _seizure or attack_

**12.** [LO 1.1] malacia
Prefix/suffix/root: _____
Definition: _softening_

**13.** [LO 1.1] plasty
Prefix/suffix/root: _____
Definition: _surgical repair_

**14.** [LO 1.1] rrhexis
Prefix/suffix/root: _____
Definition: _rupture_

**15.** [LO 1.1] tripsy
Prefix/suffix/root: _____
Definition: _surgical crushing_

**16.** [LO 1.1] uria
Prefix/suffix/root: _____
Definition: _urine or urination_

**17.** [LO 1.1] otomy
Prefix/suffix/root: _____
Definition: _to open temporarily then close_

**18.** [LO 1.1] pnea
Prefix/suffix/root: _____
Definition: _breathing_

**19.** [LO 1.1] sclerosis
Prefix/suffix/root: _____
Definition: _hardening_

**20.** [LO 1.1] stasis
Prefix/suffix/root: _____
Definition: _control or stop_

**21.** [LO 1.1] salping
Prefix/suffix/root: _____
Definition: _tube_

**22.** [LO 1.1] gastro
Prefix/suffix/root: _____
Definition: _stomach_

**23.** [LO 1.1] encephal
Prefix/suffix/root: _____
Definition: _brain_

**24.** [LO 1.1] algesi
Prefix/suffix/root: _____
Definition: _pain_

**25.** [LO 1.1] megalo
Prefix/suffix/root: _____
Definition: _large_

**26.** [LO 1.1] a
Prefix/suffix/root: _____
Definition: _____ without or absense of _____

**27.** [LO 1.1] hypo
Prefix/suffix/root: _____
Definition: _____ deficient, below _____

**28.** [LO 1.1] mono
Prefix/suffix/root: _____ one _____
Definition: _____ one _____

**29.** [LO 1.1] supra
Prefix/suffix/root: _____ above _____
Definition: _____ above _____

# Defining Medical Terms

Using your knowledge of medical definitions and word structure, define the following medical terms.

**1.** [LO 1.2] Alopecia

_____

**2.** [LO 1.2] Dermatology

_____

**3.** [LO 1.2] Intradermal

_____

**4.** [LO 1.2] Pruritis

_____

**5.** [LO 1.2] Subcutaneous

_____

**6.** [LO 1.2] Sagittal

_____

**7.** [LO 1.2] Osteorrhaphy

_____

**8.** [LO 1.2] Kyphosis

_____

**9.** [LO 1.2] Arthralgia

_____

**10.** [LO 1.2] Cardiomyopathy

_____

**11.** [LO 1.2] Cyanosis

_____

**12.** [LO 1.2] Hematoma

_____

**13.** [LO 1.2] Arteriosclerosis

_____

**14.** [LO 1.2] Aneurysm

_____

**15.** [LO 1.2] Angina

_____

## Case Studies

Read each case study below, and then answer the associated question(s).

**1.** [LO 1.2] Arthur is a diabetic patient presenting with a narrowing of the coronary arteries due to a buildup of plaque on the walls of the blood vessels. This condition is abbreviated ASHD. What does the abbreviation ASHD stand for?

_____

**2.** [LO 1.2] A history and physical is a medical document that contains a subjective history identifying the patient's chief complaint (CC), history of present illness (HPI), as well as past medical history, family, and social history (PFSH). What is the abbreviation for a history and physical as you will see it written in the patient's medical record documentation?

_____

**3.** [LO 1.2] Lucy sees her internal medicine physician for an I&D of a large abscess on her thigh. What procedure is this abbreviation commonly used to denote?

_____

**4.** [LO 1.2] You work for an endocrinologist who specializes in the treatment of diabetes. On any particular day you may see a patient with insulin-dependent diabetes mellitus. What acronym will the physician most commonly use to denote this condition?

_____

**5.** [LO 1.2] You work for Dr. Wilson, a gastroenterologist, who provides care to patients with gastroesophageal reflux disease. What is the acronym for this disease commonly seen in the medical record documentation?

_____

**6.** [LO 1.2] Amie, a medical assistant, triages a patient. During the process, the patient states, "I'm not allergic to any medications." How would Amie abbreviate this in the patient's medical record?

_____

**7.** [LO 1.1] Ms. Barker has temporal lobe epilepsy (TLE). What is the definition for the root word *lepsis*?

_____

**8.** [LO 1.1] Clarissa discovers a lump in one of her breasts and visits her physician. A screening test determines there may be a mass and her physician decides that a fine needle biopsy is required. What does the suffix *-opsy* refer to?

_____

**9.** [LO 1.1, 1.2] Irene, a 58-year-old woman with a history of smoking and a high fat diet, is admitted to the emergency room with nausea and vomiting. Women at risk for myocardial infarction can present with symptoms of nausea and vomiting; therefore, prudent cardiac protocol is followed, including CK-isoenzymes, electrocardiogram (EKG), arterial blood gases (ABGs), and complete metabolic profile (CMP).

**a.** What is the abbreviation for nausea and vomiting? _____

**b.** By breaking down the words into their component parts, what is a myocardial infarction?

_____

**10.** [LO 1.1, 1.3] Emily's primary care physician, Dr. Richards, refers her to a specialist in gastroenterology because he suspects Emily has cholecystitis. Break down the medical term *cholecystitis* into its component parts, and define the medical condition.

_____

11. [LO 1.1] Christina, a 9-year-old girl, acquires an upper respiratory infection that has resulted in inflammation of her tonsils with risk of further infection, warranting their removal. What is the medical term for the removal of tonsils?

_____

12. [LO 1.1] Carl works in the hospital laboratory and examines a variety of sputum, fecal, and blood specimens. Carl takes samples of the specimens and mounts them on slides for microscopy. Cells are examined to determine the presence or absence of disease. If disease is present, a microbiologist may analyze the specimen further to determine effective treatments. What is the medical term for the study of cells?

_____

13. [LO 1.1] Mr. Brautigan has a tube inserted into his GI tract in order to receive tube feedings, or enteral nutrition, after a severe stroke left him partially paralyzed on one side and difficulty with swallowing. What is the medical term for difficulty with swallowing?

_____

14. [LO 1.2] Sunny normally sees a naturopathic physician for herbal remedies that are not approved by the Food and Drug Administration. However, she recently developed a severe infection and agrees to conventional medical treatment. Her physician prescribes her an antibiotic medication to treat the infection. Upon receipt of the script, the pharmacy technician identifies possible contraindications between the antibiotics prescribed and the herbal remedies she takes and reports this to the head pharmacist. What is the abbreviation for the Food and Drug Administration?

_____

15. [LO 1.1] Maggie presents with malignant hypertension.
    a. What does the word part *hyper-* signify? _____
    b. What is the medical significance of the word *malignant*? _____

## Thinking It Through

Using your critical-thinking skills, answer the questions below.

1. [LO 1.3] Identify the organ system responsible for secreting hormones. List each organ involved.

_____

_____

_____

2. [LO 1.3] Describe the physiological relationship between the parathyroid gland and the bones.

_____

_____

_____

3. [LO 1.3] Explain the physiological relationship between the liver and the gallbladder.

_____

_____

_____

_____

**4.** [LO 1.3] Is there a physiological connection between the gallbladder and duodenum (first part of the small intestine)? Justify your answer.

_____

_____

_____

_____

**5.** [LO 1.3] Which body systems are affected by the relationship between the hypothalamus, pituitary gland, and the adrenal glands, commonly known as the hypothalamic-pituitary-adrenal (HPA) axis?

_____

_____

_____

_____

# 2 INTRODUCTION TO ICD-9-CM

## Learning Outcomes

*After completing this chapter, students should be able to:*

**2.1** Explain the structure of the ICD-9-CM manual.

**2.2** Describe how to use Volumes 1 and 2 to determine diagnosis codes.

**2.3** Define the conventions in Volumes 1 and 2 that help coders identify correct diagnosis codes.

**2.4** Discuss general outpatient coding principles to select appropriate diagnosis codes.

## Introduction

The diagnosis codes in the ICD-9-CM system are reported with procedure codes to indicate why a provider performed the indicated procedure. ICD-9-CM manual is divided into three volumes. The Alphabetic Index (Volume 2) is used first to locate all possible codes that may indicate the diagnosis. Those codes are then reviewed in the Tabular Index (Volume 1) to narrow the possible codes down to a single diagnosis code. Coders must use both Volume 1 and Volume 2 to determine the correct diagnosis code. ICD-9-CM Volume 3 codes are not used by coders in the physician's office. Those codes are used by hospitals to report procedures performed in the hospital.

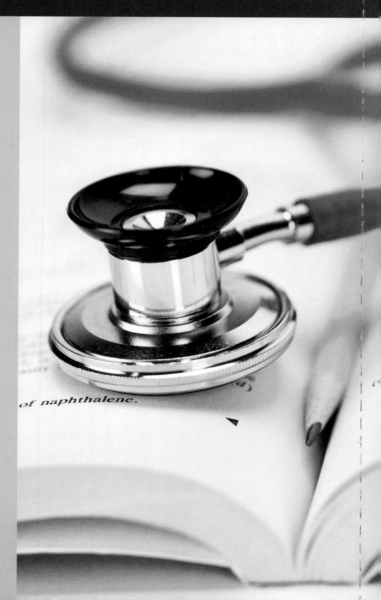

of naphthalene.

## Key Terms

Fill in each blank with the key term that best completes the sentence.

1. [LO 2.1] The _____ code set is updated each October.

2. [LO 2.1] The _____ consists of disease classification by cause and body site, supplementary classifications, and appendixes.

3. [LO 2.1] The _____ should always be used first when assigning ICD-9-CM codes.

4. [LO 2.1] Section 1 of The Alphabetic Index includes the _____ Table and Neoplasm Table.

5. [LO 2.1] The _____ includes listings for malignant, benign, and uncertain behavior.

6. [LO 2.1] The _____ includes listings for substances that may cause poisoning, by accidental or through therapeutic use.

7. [LO 2.4] The major diagnosis is usually referred to as _____ in outpatient coding.

8. [LO 2.4] The _____ is the major diagnosis in hospital coding.

9. [LO 2.4] A condition beyond the major diagnosis is known as a _____.

10. [LO 2.4] E-codes and V-codes are known as _____.

11. [LO 2.3] _____ should be used when a specific diagnosis has been made, but the codes listed do not identify the specific condition.

12. [LO 2.3] If there is not enough information to allow a specific diagnosis, the term _____ should be used.

13. [LO 2.4] _____ and symptom codes can be used when a specific diagnosis has not been made.

14. [LO 2.4] Chapter 16 of the ICD-9-CM contains many codes for _____.

15. [LO 2.4] The first-listed condition should be the major reason for a healthcare _____.

16. [LO 2.4] A subsequent _____ may have more specific details and have a more definitive diagnosis.

## Exam Review

Select the letter that best completes the statement or answers the question.

1. [LO 2.4] Diagnosis codes should be _____.
   a. As general as possible
   b. Specific regardless of whether the exact diagnosis is known
   c. Obtained only from the Alphabetic Index
   d. Reported to the highest level of specificity known

2. [LO 2.2] Which section of the ICD-9-CM should be used first to assign the appropriate diagnosis code?
   a. Volume 1, Tabular List of Diseases
   b. Volume 2, Alphabetic Index of Diseases
   c. Volume 3, Alphabetic Index and Tabular List of Procedures
   d. Appendix A

3. [LO 2.4] When coding, diagnosis codes should be listed in order of _____.
   a. Main reason for the visit listed first
   b. Alphabetic order of each diagnosis
   c. Secondary diagnosis listed first
   d. Numerical order

4. [LO 2.3] Italic brackets signify that _____.
   a. Words can be absent from a diagnosis without affecting the code to be used
   b. A modifier is needed

    **c.** A code has been revised since the previous update

    **d.** A separate code needs to be used with the diagnosis code to indicate an associated manifestation

**5.** [LO 2.3] Underlined text in the ICD-9-CM indicates _____.

    **a.** Newly added text

    **b.** New code

    **c.** Revised code

    **d.** Newly deleted text

**6.** [LO 2.3] The *5th* symbol means _____.

    **a.** A fifth digit is available as an optional selection

    **b.** A fifth digit is not available

    **c.** All codes from this selection should end in 5

    **d.** A fifth digit is necessary

**7.** [LO 2.3] The letter *M* for age conflict edits stands for _____.

    **a.** Maternity

    **b.** Mature adult

    **c.** Male between 18 and 55

    **d.** Middle aged

**8.** [LO 2.4] If a combination code is available, a coder should _____.

    **a.** Use single codes and the combination code

    **b.** Use the combination code rather than single codes

    **c.** Use single codes

    **d.** Only use if it includes a complication

**9.** [LO 2.4] If a specific diagnosis is not available after a first visit, a coder should _____.

    **a.** Not code until a diagnosis has been made

    **b.** Code for a possible diagnosis

    **c.** Code for described signs and symptoms

    **d.** Wait to code for lab results to be reported

**10.** [LO 2.4] Which of the following would be the main term to look for in the Alphabetic Index for the diagnosis "Hiatal hernia with gangrene"?

    **a.** Hiatal

    **b.** Hernia

    **c.** Gangrene

    **d.** Hiatal hernia

**11.** [LO 2.3] "Other" or "other specified" diagnosis is often indicated by a(n) _____ in the fourth digit.

    **a.** 6

    **b.** 7

    **c.** 8

    **d.** 9

**12.** [LO 2.4] A patient is seen for a routine annual checkup. What type of code should be submitted?

    **a.** Code from Volume 1 Tabular Index

    **b.** E-code

    **c.** V-code

    **d.** No code should be submitted because there was not a diagnosis.

**13.** [LO 2.3] Which fifth-digit subcategory is used when coding 250.0 for diabetes mellitus without mention of complication for type 1 not stated as uncontrolled?

    **a.** 0

    **b.** 1

**c.** 2

**d.** 3

14. [LO 2.3] Lavinia was seen for Ménière disease. The coder included code 780.4 as part of the reported diagnosis codes for dizziness. Was this code reported correctly?

    **a.** Yes, this was coded accurately.

    **b.** No, because the excludes notation mentions this disease as an exclusion.

    **c.** No, the 5th-digit notation signifies a fifth digit is needed.

    **d.** No, code 780.4 does not refer to dizziness.

15. [LO 2.3] A coder assigns diagnosis code 359.4. What else must the coder complete to code this accurately?

    **a.** Use additional E-code to identify toxic agent.

    **b.** Code first underlying disease as Addison disease 255.41.

    **c.** Required fifth digit.

    **d.** Code is correct as listed.

16. [LO 2.1] Which section of the ICD-9-CM manual is used by hospitals to identify procedures done in a facility?

    **a.** Volume 1

    **b.** Volume 2

    **c.** Volume 3

    **d.** Neoplasm Table

17. [LO 2.1] Volume 2 of the ICD-9-CM includes _____.

    **a.** Disease classification according to etiology

    **b.** Supplemental classification

    **c.** Operations on the ear

    **d.** Disease conditions and injuries along with their accompanying codes

18. [LO 2.1] The Table of Drugs and Chemicals can be found in _____.

    **a.** Volume 1

    **b.** Volume 2

    **c.** Volume 3

    **d.** Appendix A

19. [LO 2.1] The term "E-code" refers to _____.

    **a.** Codes found in the supplementary classification of external causes of injury and poisoning

    **b.** Codes found in the supplementary classification of emergency situations

    **c.** Codes found in Appendix E

    **d.** Codes found in the supplementary classification of estimation codes

20. [LO 2.1] V-codes are found in _____.

    **a.** Volume 1

    **b.** Volume 2

    **c.** Volume 3

    **d.** Appendix A

21. [LO 2.1] Volume 1 consists of _____ chapters.

    **a.** 3

    **b.** 14

    **c.** 17

    **d.** 19

22. [LO 2.1] Codes relating to mental disorders would be found in the range of _____.

    **a.** 280–289

    **b.** 290–319

    **c.** 320–389

    **d.** 780–799

23. [LO 2.1] In order to view a listing of three-digit categories, you should go to _____ in the manual.
   a. Volume 1
   b. Volume 2
   c. Appendix A
   d. Appendix E

24. [LO 2.1] Which section is found first in most ICD-9-CM manuals?
   a. Volume 1
   b. Volume 2
   c. Volume 3
   d. Table of Drugs and Chemicals

25. [LO 2.1] The most detailed information for each code can be found in _____.
   a. Volume 1
   b. Volume 2
   c. Appendixes
   d. Tables included in Volume 2

26. [LO 2.3] Using Volume 1, Tabular List of Diseases, locate code 451. What special notations are included?
   a. Includes endophlebitis
   b. Excludes that due to implant or catheter device (996.1-996.62)
   c. Uses additional E-code to identify drug, if drug induced
   d. All of the above

27. [LO 2.2] Using Volume 2, Alphabetic List of Diseases, locate *ulegyria*. What is the code associated with this term?
   a. 523.8
   b. 533.8
   c. 742.4
   d. 724.4

28. [LO 2.1] Using the Table of Drugs and Chemicals, what code is listed for poisoning by Epsom salt?
   a. 971.2
   b. 973.3
   c. E858.4
   d. 962.0

29. [LO 2.2] Using Volume 1, find the V-code V70. What fourth digit should be used for an unspecified general medical examination?
   a. 0
   b. 2
   c. 8
   d. 9

30. [LO 2.2] Using Volume 2, Index to External Causes, locate the external cause cut by ice pick. What E-code is listed?
   a. E920.4
   b. E920.3
   c. E924.0
   d. 920.4

## Navigating the ICD Manual

Using your ICD manual, complete each sentence below.

1. [LO 2.1] Physicians and other professionals do not use codes from _____ to report procedures.

2. [LO 2.1] Chapters in Volume 1 cover codes describing _____.

3. [LO 2.1] Section 1 of Volume 2 includes the _____ and _____ Tables.

4. [LO 2.1] The _____ includes extensive lists of drugs, industrial solvents, noxious plants, pesticides, and other toxic agents.

5. [LO 2.1] V-codes are found in _____.

6. [LO 2.1] _____ include codes with a fourth or fourth and fifth digit to report the diagnosis in more detail.

7. [LO 2.1] E-codes and V-codes are known as _____.

8. [LO 2.1] Volume 1 includes _____ appendixes.

9. [LO 2.1] A coder should use the _____ to locate the accurate code for a benign tumor of the rectosigmoid junction.

10. [LO 2.4] A coder reporting an injury from a fall from a ladder should assign the appropriate _____.

11. [LO 2.1] The hypertension table includes the _____, _____, and _____ categories.

12. [LO 2.4] _____ should be used for patients that are seen for an annual checkup.

13. [LO 2.1] Volume 1 of the ICD-9-CM may include common code designations at the _____ of the code section.

14. [LO 2.3] Code 372.39 Pingueculitis includes a notation that excludes _____.

15. [LO 2.3] Code 656.3 Fetal distress requires a _____.

## Thinking It Through

Using your critical-thinking skills, answer the following questions.

1. [LO 2.1] Who currently maintains and publishes updates to ICD-9-CM?

_____

_____

_____

2. [LO 2.2] Why should a coder not rely only on the Alphabetic Index to determine the appropriate code for a diagnosis?

_____

_____

_____

3. [LO 2.3] If a code has 5th digit notation in the tabular list, is it acceptable to list only four digits? Why or why not?

_____

_____

_____

4. [LO 2.3] Locate the term *organic* in the Alphabetic Index. What notations are listed?

_____

_____

_____

5. [LO 2.3] A coder submits code 530.4 for a traumatic perforation of esophagus. Is this acceptable? Explain why or why not?

_____

_____

_____

# 3

# ICD-9-CM CHAPTER-SPECIFIC GUIDELINES, PART I: CHAPTERS 1–10

## Learning Outcomes

*After completing this chapter, students should be able to:*

**3.1** Identify the most appropriate diagnosis codes to report infectious and parasitic diseases; neoplasms; endocrine, nutritional, and metabolic diseases; and immunity system disorders.

**3.2** Recognize diagnosis codes for diseases of blood and blood-forming organs; mental

disorders; and disorders of the nervous system and sense organs.

**3.3** Name the correct diagnosis codes to describe diseases of the circulatory and respiratory systems.

**3.4** List diagnosis codes for diseases of the digestive and genitourinary systems.

## Introduction

This chapter begins the review of the ICD-9-CM coding system, including ICD-9-CM chapters 1–10. Specific topics covered by these ICD-9-CM chapters include infectious diseases (Chapter 1); neoplasms (Chapter 2); endocrine, nutritional, metabolic, and immunity disorders (Chapter 3); diseases of blood and blood-forming organs (Chapter 4); mental disorders (Chapter 5); nervous system and sense organs (Chapter 6); circulatory system (Chapter 7); respiratory system (Chapter 8); digestive system (Chapter 9); and genitourinary system (Chapter 10). Each chapter in the ICD-9-CM manual includes explanations of the chapter-specific guidance.

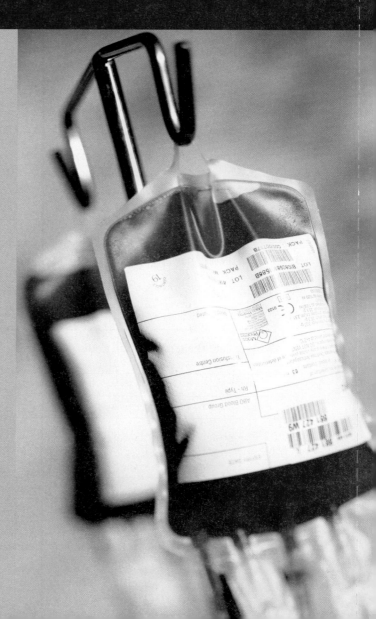

## Key Terms

Fill in the blanks with the key term that most accurately matches the description.

1. _____ Decreased insulin production usually beginning in childhood
2. _____ Stroke or cerebrovascular accident
3. _____ High blood pressure
4. _____ Chronic deteriorating condition of lungs
5. _____ Medical terminology for new growth
6. _____ Blood poisoning, caused by microorganisms in blood
7. _____ Adult-onset condition with decreased response to insulin and elevated glucose
8. _____ Neoplasm at its place of origin
9. _____ Staph infection that is resistant to certain antibiotics
10. _____ Long-term renal illness
11. _____ Active infection with human immunodeficiency virus
12. _____ Infection with HIV virus without any symptoms—code as V08
13. _____ Origin of cancer cells or malignancies
14. _____ Elevated glucose caused by illness or pregnancy
15. _____ Symptoms include tachycardia, fever, tachypnea, leukocytosis
16. _____ First site of cancer location, first-listed diagnosis
17. _____ May be metastasis or second site of cancer, supplemental diagnosis
18. _____ Chronic kidney failure severe enough to require dialysis
19. _____ Another term related to cancerous cells
20. _____ Secondary illness caused by compromised immune system due to HIV status

## Exam Review

Select the letter that best describes the statement or answers the question.

1. [LO 3.3] Which specific types of hypertension are included in the Hypertension Table?
   a. Malignant, benign, unspecified
   b. Primary, secondary, tertiary
   c. Essential, transient, orthostatic
   d. Unspecified, hypertensive, diabetic

2. [LO.3.2] A 70-year-old left-handed man with right-sided hemiparesis and aphasia due to a previous left cerebral stroke has new onset of an acute right-sided CVA with cerebral infarction. These conditions are indicated with the following codes:
   a. 434.91, 438.20, 438.11
   b. 434.01, 438.11, 438.21
   c. 434.91, 438.11, 438.22
   d. 437.0, 438.11, 438.20

3. [LO 3.1] A patient is admitted to the hospital for a surgery to excise a metastatic tumor in the liver. The primary tumor is located in the hilum of the lung and cannot be removed surgically. Immediately following surgery, the patient receives chemotherapy to treat the tumor. What diagnosis codes would the treating physicians report?
   a. 197.7, 162.2, V58.11
   b. 162.2, 197.7, V58.11
   c. 197.0, 197.7, V58.11
   d. 197.7, 155.2, V58.11

**4.** [LO 3.1]  A physician sees a patient with septicemia due to anthrax. What code is used to identify this condition?

   **a.** 038.40

   **b.** 038.9

   **c.** 022.3

   **d.** 995.91

**5.** [LO 3.4]  Using the Tabular Listing of Diseases, identify which system is described by codes in Chapter 10.

   **a.** Endocrine, nutritional, and metabolic diseases

   **b.** Genitourinary system

   **c.** Congenital anomalies

   **d.** Pulmonary system

**6.** [LO 3.1]  A physician sees a patient in his office to follow up on a positive HIV test. The patient is asymptomatic with no known HIV-related conditions. What diagnosis code is used to identify the patient's HIV status?

   **a.** 042

   **b.** V08

   **c.** 042 as the first-listed code plus additional codes to identify possible HIV-related conditions

   **d.** V01.89 and 042

**7.** [LO 3.1]  When coding for SIRS, what are the guidelines?

   **a.** Always use two codes—one for the underlying cause and another for the subcategory.

   **b.** Always code the subcategory first and the underlying cause second.

   **c.** (*a*) and (*b*)

   **d.** Neither (*a*) or (*b*)

**8.** [LO 3.1]  When coding for MRSA, what are the guidelines?

   **a.** It will always be a combination code that includes the infective agent.

   **b.** It will always be two separate codes: one for infection and one for agent.

   **c.** It can be either combination or multiple codes, depending on situation.

   **d.** None of the above.

**9.** [LO 3.2]  What are the criteria when coding for pain?

   **a.** Pain codes are always primary in nature.

   **b.** Pain codes are always secondary to the disease state.

   **c.** Pain codes in 338 range can either be primary or secondary depending on the reason the patient is seen by the physician.

   **d.** Pain codes are a separate category and are neither primary nor secondary.

**10.** [LO 3.3]  When would you use code 496 when treating COPD?

   **a.** This is a nonspecific code and is only used if the level of diagnosis is not specified.

   **b.** This will always be the first-listed diagnosis code when coding for COPD.

   **c.** When asthmatic conditions are involved.

   **d.** Never.

**11.** [LO 3.1, 3.3]  When coding for chronic kidney disease with diabetes, which code goes first?

   **a.** Chronic kidney disease is coded first as first-listed diagnosis.

   **b.** Diabetes is coded first as first-listed diagnosis.

   **c.** It would depend on stage of kidney disease.

   **d.** It is reported as a combination code.

**12.** [LO 3.1, 3.3]  Where does the code for HIV go on an HIV-positive patient being seen for an illness unrelated to HIV?

   **a.** HIV is always the primary code as underlying illness.

   **b.** HIV would not be coded as the illness is unrelated.

   **c.** HIV would be the secondary code, and illness would be coded as primary.

   **d.** None of the above.

**13.** [LO 3.1] A patient is seen by her physician to evaluate her type II diabetes that requires regular use of insulin. She also has stage III renal failure and controlled hypertension secondary to her diabetes. Which of the following are the appropriate codes to report these conditions, including the correct order of the codes?

   **a.** 250.4, 405.11, 585.3
   **b.** 250.40, 403.10, 585.3, V58.67
   **c.** 585.3, 403.10, 250.40
   **d.** 403.10, 585.3, 250.40, V58.67

**14.** [LO 3.3] A pediatrician sees a patient with asthma. The child had been stable on his medications, but over the last week has had an acute exacerbation of his disease, which has now progressed to status asthmaticus. This condition would be described by code(s) _____.

   **a.** 493.0
   **b.** 493.02, 493.01
   **c.** 493.01
   **d.** 493.02

**15.** [LO 3.1, 3.2] Which additional code is used to indicate the cause of an injury when a patient presents with an injury that is related to an external cause?

   **a.** V-code
   **b.** Neoplasm code
   **c.** E-code
   **d.** NEC-code

**16.** [LO 3.1] Chronic condition of tonsils and adenoids due to secondary diabetes would be reported as _____.

   **a.** 249.3, 731.8
   **b.** 249.9, 785.4
   **c.** 474, 249.2
   **d.** 474.12, 249.8

**17.** [LO 3.1] Diabetic cataract due to uncontrolled type II diabetes would be reported as _____.

   **a.** 250.01, 366.4
   **b.** 250.02, 366.41
   **c.** 366.4, 250.02
   **d.** 250.02, 366.4

**18.** [LO 3.1] Empyema due to MRSA would be reported as _____.

   **a.** 510, 041.12
   **b.** 510.9, 041.12
   **c.** 041.12, 510
   **d.** 041.11, 510.9

**19.** [LO 3.1, 3.4] Crigler-Najjar disease/syndrome would be reported as _____.

   **a.** 277.06
   **b.** 315.9
   **c.** 277.4
   **d.** 208.1

**20.** [LO 3.4] Primary malignant neoplasms of the femur would be reported as _____.

   **a.** 198.5
   **b.** 170.7
   **c.** 165.8
   **d.** 170.8

**21.** [LO 3.4] Prenatal care during first pregnancy complicated by hypertensive kidney disease would be reported as _____.

   **a.** 642.23
   **b.** 642.20, V22.2

   **c.** V22.1, 642.23

   **d.** 642.20, V22.0

**22.** [LO 3.4] GERD (gastroesophageal reflux disorder) would be reported as _____.

   **a.** 530.8

   **b.** 530.81

   **c.** 530.82

   **d.** 530.08

**23.** [LO 3.1] Septic shock would be reported as _____.

   **a.** 785.52

   **b.** 785.25

   **c.** 587.25

   **d.** 584.5

**24.** [LO 3.1] Personal history of MRSA (methicillin-resistant *Staphylococcus aureus*) would be reported as _____.

   **a.** 041.12

   **b.** V02.54

   **c.** V12.04

   **d.** V12.04, 041.12

**25.** [LO 3.1] Hashimoto thyroiditis would be reported as _____.

   **a.** 254.20

   **b.** 245.2

   **c.** 245.9

   **d.** 245.21

**26.** [LO 3.1, 3.3] Primary tracheobronchial tuberculosis. Bacilli are found in the sputum. This would be reported as _____.

   **a.** 010.83

   **b.** 011.90

   **c.** 011.33

   **d.** 012.33

**27.** [LO 3.1] Exophthalmic goiter with thyrotoxic storm would be reported as _____.

   **a.** 242.0

   **b.** 242.00

   **c.** 242.01

   **d.** 240.9

**28.** [LO 3.2, 3.4] Cirrhosis of liver associated with alcoholism would be reported as _____.

   **a.** 571.5

   **b.** 571.2

   **c.** 571.52

   **d.** 571.0

**29.** [LO 3.2] Senile dementia with acute confused state would be reported as _____.

   **a.** 294.8

   **b.** 290.0

   **c.** 290.3

   **d.** 295.00

**30.** [LO 3.4] Diverticulitis of colon with hemorrhage would be reported as _____.

   **a.** 562.10

   **b.** 562.11

   **c.** 562.12

   **d.** 562.13

# Applying Your Skills

Using your ICD-9-CM manual, assign the correct code(s) for each diagnosis.

1. [LO 3.1] Diabetes mellitus type I, controlled. _____

    (ICD-10-CM: _____)

2. [LO 3.1] Diabetes mellitus type II, uncontrolled. _____

    (ICD-10-CM: _____)

3. [LO 3.1] Gestational diabetes, controlled. _____

    (ICD-10-CM: _____)

4. [LO 3.1] Neoplasm, benign, great toe. _____

    (ICD-10-CM: _____)

5. [LO 3.1] Neoplasm, lung, malignant, primary. _____

    (ICD-10-CM: _____)

6. [LO 3.3] Hypertension benign. _____

    (ICD-10-CM: _____)

7. [LO 3.3] Malignant hypertension. _____

    (ICD-10-CM: _____)

8. [LO 3.2] Septicemia. _____

    (ICD-10-CM: _____)

9. [LO 3.2] Septic shock. _____

    (ICD-10-CM: _____)

10. [LO 3.1] HIV. _____

    (ICD-10-CM: _____)

11. [LO 3.3] CVA. _____

    (ICD-10-CM: _____)

12. [LO 3.1] MRSA, wound, open, hand. _____

    (ICD-10-CM: _____)

13. [LO 3.4] End-stage renal disease. _____

    (ICD-10-CM: _____)

14. [LO 3.4] Stage I chronic kidney disease. _____

    (ICD-10-CM: _____)

15. [LO 3.1] Kaposi sarcoma of skin of face. _____

    (ICD-10-CM: _____)

# Case Studies

Read each case study. Assign the ICD-9-CM code(s) to accurately describe each scenario, and answer the associated questions.

1. [LO 3.1] A 22-year-old male is admitted to the hospital with chronic tonsillitis, HIV, and Kaposi sarcoma of the lymph nodes. Code all his conditions.

    _____

    (ICD-10-CM: _____)

**2.** [LO 3.1, 3.4] Mrs. Reese, a 33-year-old woman, presents to ER after exposure to smallpox in Nigeria. Code the diagnosis only.

_____

(ICD-10-CM: _____)

**3.** [LO 3.1] A 12-year-old boy presents to the emergency clinic with diagnosis of malarial hepatitis. Please list the two codes, and identify which is the first-listed diagnosis and which is the secondary. How did you identify the secondary diagnosis?

_____

_____

(ICD-10-CM: _____)

**4.** [LO 3.4] A 45-year-old man presents to a proctologist complaining of thrombosed external hemorrhoids and ulcerated internal hemorrhoids.

_____

(ICD-10-CM: _____)

**5.** [LO 3.2] Ms. Prescott is admitted to the psychiatric unit with mixed diagnosis of obsessive-compulsive disorder, panic attack, and psychasthenic episode.

_____

(ICD-10-CM: _____)

**6.** [LO 3.2] A 21-year-old man presents to the emergency room after an altercation in a bar. He presents with a complicated wound of eyebrow, multiple wounds to lower leg, closed fracture of the shaft of the radius, and a closed fracture of the skull. He denies loss of consciousness. Code the diagnoses in order of severity.

_____

(ICD-10-CM: _____)

**7.** [LO 3.1] Wendy presents for her routine postpartum visit and to follow up for a uterine tumor found during delivery. Provide both codes.

_____

(ICD-10-CM: _____)

**8.** [LO 3.4, 3.2] A 55-year-old man is admitted to ICU with diagnoses of hepatitis B with hepatic coma, alcoholic cirrhosis, and hepatomegaly. Provide all three codes.

_____

(ICD-10-CM: _____)

**9.** [LO 3.1] Stewart presents to his family physician requesting screening blood testing for measles, whooping cough, and rubella.

_____

(ICD-10-CM: _____)

**10.** [LO 3.1] Colin returned from spring break and presented to his dermatologist complaining of tinea capitis, tinea corporis, tinea cruris, and pediculosis infestation. Provide all four codes.

_____

_____

(ICD-10-CM: _____)

Define tinea capitis: _____

Define tinea corporis:_____

Define tinea cruris: _____

Define pediculosis: _____

**11.** [LO 3.1] Mr. Long presented to the emergency department with urticaria caused by foods he ingested at lunch.

_____

(ICD-10-CM: _____)

**12.** [LO 3.4] An elderly patient presents to her urologist with nocturia, enuresis, hematuria, and dysuria. Provide all four codes.

_____

(ICD-10-CM: _____)

**13.** [LO 3.2] Corrine presents to the emergency department with exacerbation of her microcytic hypochromic anemia due to chronic blood loss.

_____

(ICD-10-CM: _____)

**14.** [LO 3.1] A 35-year-old woman presents to an endocrinologist after diagnosis of systemic lupus erythematosus.

_____

(ICD-10-CM: _____)

**15.** [LO 3.1] A patient presents to the ophthalmologist with diabetic retinopathy and malignant myopia, secondary to uncontrolled type I diabetes. Provide all three codes.

_____

(ICD-10-CM: _____)

## Thinking It Through

Using your critical-thinking skills, answer the following questions.

**1.** [LO 3.2] What are the three types of pain covered under code 338? What is the designation for the pain code in order to be considered under code 338? Are you able to designate code 338 if pain is due to underlying illness or disease state? Why or why not?

_____

_____

_____

_____

**2.** [LO 3.2, 3.4] When coding for anemia resulting from other chronic disease, what is the coding process when anemia is the cause for the visit? What would be the coding process if an underlying disease is the cause for the visit?

_____

_____

_____

_____

**3.** [LO 3.4] List the stages of renal disease. When you are coding for ESRD, what are two other diseases that are considered common contributing factors? How would you code the case of a patient, on dialysis, who has end-stage renal disease and anemia?

_____

_____

_____

_____

**4.** [LO 3.2, 3.4] A patient is diagnosed with the following conditions: B complex deficiency, osteomalacia, and adult failure to thrive due to anorexia nervosa. List the codes for these diagnoses. Identify which code would be listed first, and why.

_____

_____

_____

_____

**5.** [LO 3.1, 3.2] If a patient is diagnosed with acute megakaryocytic leukemia in relapse with acquired aplastic anemia due to antineoplastic chemotherapy, how would you code both conditions in appropriate order (with the M-code for leukemia)?

_____

_____

_____

_____

# ICD-9-CM CHAPTER-SPECIFIC GUIDELINES, PART II: CHAPTERS 11–19

## Learning Outcomes

*After completing this chapter, students should be able to:*

**4.1** Select appropriate diagnosis codes describing complications of pregnancy, childbirth, and the puerperium.

**4.2** Identify codes for diseases of the skin and of subcutaneous, musculoskeletal, and connective tissues.

**4.3** Identify diagnosis codes describing congenital anomalies; newborn (perinatal) condition guidelines; signs, symptoms, and ill-defined conditions; and injuries and poisonings.

**4.4** Describe the uses of E-codes and V-codes.

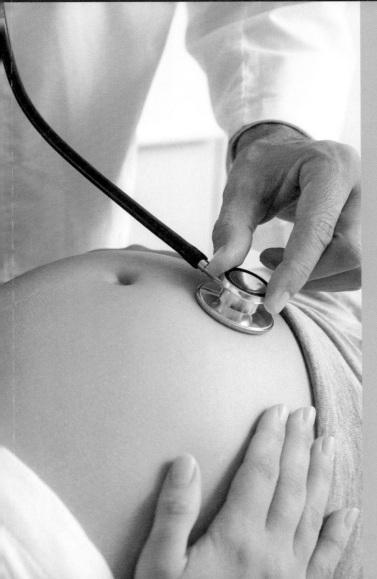

## Introduction

This chapter completes the review of the ICD-9-CM coding system, including ICD-9-CM chapters 11–19. Specific topics covered by these ICD-9-CM chapters include pregnancy, childbirth, and the puerperium (Chapter 11); the skin and sub-cutaneous tissue (Chapter 12); musculoskeletal and connective tissue (Chapter 13); congenital anomalies (Chapter 14); conditions originating in the perinatal period (Chapter 15); signs, symptoms, and ill-defined conditions (Chapter 16); and injury and poisoning (Chapter 17). In addition to completing the review of specific disease-oriented chapters (Chapters 11–17), the supplemental classification codes are covered, including V-codes (Chapter 18) and E-codes (Chapter 19). The discussion of each chapter of the ICD-9-CM manual includes an explanation of the chapter-specific guidance included in that chapter.

# Key Terms

Fill in each blank with the key term that best completes the sentence.

1. [LO 4.1] Sites for a(n) _____ include abdominal, tubal, and ovarian.

2. [LO 4.1] Ectopic and _____ can be found in the subchapter 630–633.

3. [LO 4.3] The _____ period usually lasts between three and six weeks.

4. [LO 4.4] Normal _____ are coded with V22.0 or V22.1.

5. [LO 4.1] A patient that has a(n) _____ should have the condition that resulted in the admission as the first-listed diagnosis.

6. [LO 4.1] _____ can increase the risk for developing diabetes later.

7. [LO 4.1] Immediately following delivery until six weeks following delivery is known as the _____.

8. [LO 4.1] The _____ begins in the last month of pregnancy and lasts for five months after delivery.

9. [LO 4.2] Severe osteoporosis can lead to _____.

10. [LO 4.3] _____ are conditions that are present at birth.

11. [LO 4.4] If a patient requires continued care throughout the recovery or healing process, a(n) _____ code should be assigned.

# Exam Review

Select the letter that best completes each statement or question

1. [LO 4.1, 4.2, 4.3, 4.4] If a fourth- or fifth-digit requirement applies to multiple categories or subcategories, it is noted with _____.
   a. Bracketed listing of which digits can be used
   b. Bulleted listing with indicators of which fourth or fifth digit can be used
   c. Appropriate fourth or fifth digits are listed above the code
   d. Red parentheses that appear after the code with indicators of which fourth or fifth digit can be used

2. [LO 4.1] When coding for a diagnosis of a patient who is pregnant, but was seen for reasons not relating to the pregnancy, which V-code should be used?
   a. V22.0
   b. V22.1
   c. V22.2
   d. V23

3. [LO 4.1] An admission that results in a delivery must include a V-code to describe the _____.
   a. Length of labor
   b. Age of mother
   c. Pain medication administered
   d. Type of delivery

4. [LO 4.1] A woman is diagnosed with gestational diabetes. The codes reported are 648.0 and 648.8. Is this correct?
   a. Yes, this is correct.
   b. No, code 250 should also be reported.
   c. No, only code 648.0 is required.
   d. No, codes 648.0 and 648.8 are never reported together.

5. [LO 4.4] What is the only V-code that is appropriate to use with code 650?
   a. V22.0
   b. V22.1
   c. V27.0
   d. V27.1

**6.** [LO 4.2] Codes from subcategory 733.1 are used to report _____ for a pathological fracture.

  **a.** Active treatment
  **b.** Aftercare
  **c.** Past history
  **d.** Family history

**7.** [LO 4.3] Codes from Chapter 14, congenital abnormalities, _____.

  **a.** Are only used at birth
  **b.** Can be reported from birth to 1 year of age.
  **c.** Can be reported throughout a patient's lifetime
  **d.** Cannot be reported at birth

**8.** [LO 4.1, 4.2, 4.3] A condition that requires increased nursing care is _____.

  **a.** Community acquired
  **b.** Clinically insignificant
  **c.** Clinically significant
  **d.** Hospital acquired

**9.** [LO 4.3] When multiple injuries are present, _____.

  **a.** The most serious injury is the only one coded
  **b.** All injuries are coded separately
  **c.** Superficial injuries such as contusions are coded
  **d.** Categories describing combinations of injuries cannot be used

**10.** [LO 4.3] When coding for a burn, the total body surface area (BSA) percentage for an adult having a burn of the upper extremities is _____.

  **a.** 1          **c.** 14
  **b.** 9          **d.** 18

**11.** [LO 4.4] V-codes _____.

  **a.** Cannot be used in a hospital setting
  **b.** Can only be secondary diagnosis codes
  **c.** Can be either a primary or secondary diagnosis code
  **d.** Cannot be used for aftercare

**12.** [LO 4.4] A patient that has been seen because of contact with a communicable disease should _____.

  **a.** Be coded with V-code V01
  **b.** Be coded with V-code V70.0
  **c.** Be coded with the corresponding code to the disease
  **d.** Not have any code listed

**13.** [LO 4.4] E-codes _____.

  **a.** Are only used for poisoning
  **b.** Can be used as the first-listed diagnosis
  **c.** Cannot be used as the first-listed diagnosis
  **d.** Are only used for accidents that occur outside the home

**14.** [LO 4.2] When coding for a pressure ulcer, _____.

  **a.** Only the code 707.0 is needed
  **b.** Code 707.0 and a code for the location are needed
  **c.** Code 707.0 and a code for the stage are needed
  **d.** Only the code 707.2 is needed

**15.** [LO 4.4] If a patient has a parent that is deaf _____.

  **a.** No code should be assigned
  **b.** Code V19.2 should be assigned
  **c.** Code 389.9 should be used
  **d.** Code V19.2 and 398.9 should be used

**16.** [LO 4.1]  What is the code for severe preeclampsia?

    **a.** 642.5

    **b.** 642.50

    **c.** 642.6

    **d.** 642.3

**17.** [LO 4.1]  Following labor and delivery, Mrs. Barnes experienced acute kidney failure. What is the code for this as a postpartum condition?

    **a.** 584.9

    **b.** 586

    **c.** 669.31

    **d.** 669.34

**18.** [LO 4.2]  What is the code for ammonia dermatitis?

    **a.** 691

    **b.** 691.0

    **c.** 692.9

    **d.** 983.2

**19.** [LO 4.2]  What is the code for a pressure ulcer with full thickness skin loss located on the ankle?

    **a.** 707.06

    **b.** 707.06, 707.23

    **c.** 707.13

    **d.** 707.13, 707.23

**20.** [LO 4.2]  What is the code for Baastrup syndrome?

    **a.** 695.19

    **b.** 721.5

    **c.** 721.52

    **d.** 721.42

**21.** [LO 4.3]  What is the code for spina bifida of the lumbar region?

    **a.** 741

    **b.** 741.3

    **c.** 741.93

    **d.** 756.17

**22.** [LO 4.3]  What is the code for phrenic nerve paralysis?

    **a.** 799.21

    **b.** 767.7

    **c.** 354.8

    **d.** 767.5

**23.** [LO 4.3]  Penny presents with a high fever. What is the code for this sign?

    **a.** 780.60

    **b.** 780.6

    **c.** 778.4

    **d.** 780.64

**24.** [LO 4.3]  What is the code for closed dislocation of the shoulder?

    **a.** 831.00

    **b.** 831.9

    **c.** 718.31

    **d.** 831.10

25. [LO 4.3]  What is the code for poisoning by vitamin K?
    a. 934.3
    b. 858.2
    c. 964.3
    d. 950.4

26. [LO 4.4]  What code should be used for a personal history of malignant neoplasm of the bone?
    a. V10.81
    b. V10.91
    c. V10.90
    d. 170.9

27. [LO 4.4]  Annabelle is 15 years old and is admitted to the hospital as a high-risk pregnancy. What is the code?
    a. V22.0
    b. V23.83
    c. V23.89
    d. V23.9

28. [LO 4.4]  Dr. Gabreski recommends HIV counseling to a patient. What is the code for human immunodeficiency virus (HIV) counseling?
    a. V65.44
    b. V65.40
    c. V65.49
    d. V65.4

29. [LO 4.4]  An injury received when sewing would be reported as _____.
    a. E018.0
    b. E12.0
    c. E12.1
    d. E12.0

30. [LO 4.4]  An accidental poisoning by antibiotics would be reported as _____.
    a. E856
    b. E858.9
    c. E930.9
    d. E950.4

## Applying Your Skills

Using your ICD-9-CM manual, assign the correct code(s) for each diagnosis.

1. [LO 4.1]  Mrs. Sanchez suffers a hemorrhage at 19 weeks of gestation. _____
   (ICD-10-CM: _____)

2. [LO 4.1]  Patient presents with anemia at 33 weeks gestation. _____
   (ICD-10-CM: _____)

3. [LO 4.2]  Bill presents with paronychia of the finger after swimming. _____
   (ICD-10-CM: _____)

4. [LO 4.2]  Contact dermatitis due to exposure to iodine. _____
   (ICD-10-CM: _____)

5. [LO 4.2]  Rheumatoid arthritis. _____
   (ICD-10-CM: _____)

6. [LO 4.3]  Unilateral complete cleft lip. _____
   (ICD-10-CM: _____)

**7.** [LO 4.3] A newborn requires aspiration. _____

(ICD-10-CM: _____)

**8.** [LO 4.3] Jesse is 5 years old and is described as having failure to thrive. _____

(ICD-10-CM: _____)

**9.** [LO 4.3] After an automobile accident, Maria presents with a heart (myocardial) contusion. _____

(ICD-10-CM: _____)

**10.** [LO 4.3} Zachary is poisoned by antiasthmatics. _____

(ICD-10-CM: _____)

**11.** [LO 4.4] Prescription of oral contraceptives. _____

(ICD-10-CM: _____)

**12.** [LO 4.4] Convalescence and palliative care following chemotherapy. _____

(ICD-10-CM: _____)

**13.** [LO 4.4] Stephen is assaulted by another boy with a BB gun. _____

(ICD-10-CM: _____)

**14.** [LO 4.4] While racing in the Belmont Stakes, Elizabeth fell from her horse. _____

(ICD-10-CM: _____)

**15.** [LO 4.4] Mr. O'Connor was birdwatching in a field when he was suddenly struck by lightning. _____

(ICD-10-CM: _____)

## Case Studies

For each of the following scenarios, assign the appropriate ICD-9-CM code(s).

**1.** [LO 4.1] A female patient presents with acute pelvic pain and vaginal bleeding. A pregnancy test is performed with a positive result. After a pelvic exam and ultrasound, it is determined that the patient is suffering from an ectopic pregnancy in the fallopian tube without intrauterine pregnancy. Endometriosis was discovered. _____

(ICD-10-CM: _____)

**2.** [LO 4.2] A patient brings his 9-month-old son to the doctor's office because he has noticed yellowish scales on the infant's head. A physical exam is completed, and the doctor diagnoses the infant with cradle cap.

_____

(ICD-10-CM: _____)

**3.** [LO 4.2] A patient complains of pain and stiffness of the fingers. After a physical examination has been completed, the doctor orders a blood test. Results are returned stating a positive rheumatoid factor and elevated ESR. The doctor diagnoses rheumatoid arthritis and states that it is polyneuropathic. _____

(ICD-10-CM: _____)

**4.** [LO 4.3] A 3-month-old child is brought to the doctor because of an enlarged head and bulging eyes. A skull x-ray and angiography are ordered. The child is diagnosed with hydrocephalus. _____

(ICD-10-CM: _____)

**5.** [LO 4.3] A patient in her seventh month of pregnancy presents with bright red vaginal bleeding. A pelvic ultrasound is completed, and the mother is diagnosed with placenta previa.

(ICD-10-CM: _____)

**6.** [LO 4.3] A patient presents with a persistent headache. After an examination, no illness was detected. Patient was prescribed medication to assist with the pain and directed to return in a week if still experiencing the symptom.

_____

(ICD-10-CM: _____)

7. [LO 4.3, 4.4] A patient was seen that had fallen from a ladder while cleaning gutters at home. The patient lost consciousness for a period of time. The patient now has a headache and blurred vision. An x-ray was ordered, and it was found that the patient was suffering from a concussion. _____

   (ICD-10-CM: _____)

8. [LO 4.4] A newborn is seen at the doctor's at 2 weeks of age for a weight check to make sure he is receiving adequate nutrition through breast feeding. _____

   (ICD-10-CM: _____)

9. [LO 4.3, 4.4] A patient presents with a swollen ankle that occurred during a rugby game. It is determined by a physical exam and x-ray to be a sprained ankle. _____

   (ICD-10-CM: _____)

10. [LO 4.3, 4.4] A patient is seen by the doctor after falling and cutting her knee on glass. _____

    (ICD-10-CM: _____)

## Thinking It Through

Using your critical-thinking skills, answer the following questions.

1. [LO 4.1, 4.4] Describe the usual method of coding for obstetric care.

   _____

   _____

   _____

   _____

2. [LO 4.3] When can congenital abnormalities be reported? Why?

   _____

   _____

   _____

   _____

3. [LO 4.3] Describe the use of the Table of Drugs and Chemicals.

   _____

   _____

   _____

   _____

4. [LO 4.3] What is the process for coding a burn?

   _____

   _____

   _____

   _____

5. [LO 4.4] When should the code E849.9 be used?

   _____

   _____

   _____

   _____

# 5 INTRODUCTION TO ICD-10-CM AND ICD-10-PCS

## Learning Outcomes

*After completing this chapter, students should be able to:*

**5.1** Describe the upcoming transition to ICD-10-CM.

**5.2** Discuss the basic structure of ICD-10-CM diagnosis codes.

**5.3** Explain the structure of the ICD-10-CM manual.

**5.4** Compare ICD-10-CM general guidelines with ICD-9-CM guidelines.

**5.5** Discuss the structure of the ICD-10-PCS system for procedure codes.

## Introduction

The ICD-10-CM diagnosis coding system will be implemented on October 1, 2013. As the implementation date approaches, coders must both know the ICD-9-CM system in detail and become knowledgeable about ICD-10-CM codes. This chapter outlines the similarities and differences between the two coding systems.

One of the major differences between the ICD-9-CM and ICD-10-CM coding systems is that the ICD-9-CM includes both diagnosis and procedure codes. ICD-10-CM only includes diagnosis codes. Procedure codes are included in the ICD-10-PCS coding system, which will be used by hospitals to report procedures performed in the hospital setting. Another difference is that the new ICD-10-CM codes are up to seven digits in length.

The ICD-10-CM manual is divided into 21 chapters, 2 more than the current ICD-9-CM diagnosis code chapters. The new chapters list specific diagnoses involving the eye and the ear. The order of the chapters has been revised so that related chapters are grouped together. Some of the coding conventions and symbols used in the ICD-10-CM manual have also been revised from those used in the ICD-9-CM manual.

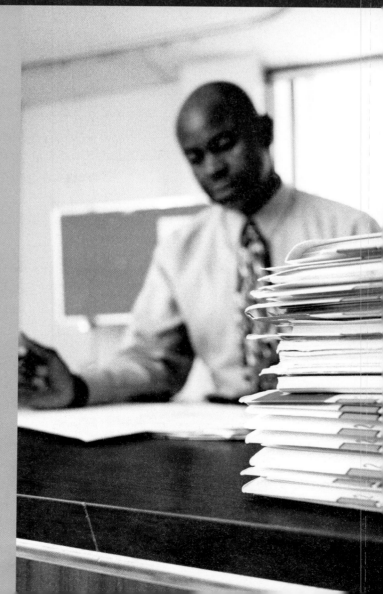

# Key Terms

Fill in each blank with the key term that best completes the sentence.

1. [LO 5.4] The _____ note is used to signify that the diagnostic terms listed after the note are not part of the condition(s), "Not included here."

2. [LO 5.4] "Not coded here" indicates that the code excluded should never be used at the same time as the code above the _____ note.

3. [LO 5.2] The term _____ describes which side of the body the condition or specific site is located.

4. [LO 5.5] Inpatient facility procedures are coded using _____.

5. [LO 5.2] ICD-10-CM uses a(n) _____ character, _____, to allow for future expansion.

6. [LO 5.4] A sign of a disease is the _____.

7. [LO 5.4] _____ is the study of causes of diseases.

8. [LO 5.4] The _____ note tells you it is acceptable to use both code and the excluded code together when both conditions exist.

9. [LO 5.2] Late effects of an injury or illness are also known in ICD-10-CM as _____.

10. [LO 5.1] To help crosswalk ICD-9 codes to ICD-10 codes, a(n) _____ was developed.

# Exam Review

Select the letter that best completes each statement or question.

1. [LO 5.3] The primary arrangement for diagnoses in the index is _____.
   a. Location
   b. Severity
   c. Site
   d. Condition

2. [LO 5.2] An "x" in the fifth and sixth position is used to indicate _____.
   a. An unspecified site
   b. An "NOS" condition
   c. A placeholder between two valid characters
   d. Bilateral condition

3. [LO 5.2] ICD-10-CM codes consist of _____.
   a. Five to seven digits
   b. Three to eight digits
   c. Three to seven digits
   d. Three to five digits

4. [LO 5.2] The initial treatment is indicated by adding a character to the _____.
   a. Third digit
   b. Seventh digit
   c. Fifth digit
   d. Eighth digit

5. [LO 5.2] The first character of ICD-10-CM _____.
   a. Is always a number
   b. Can be either a number or letter
   c. Is always a letter
   d. Is none of these

6. [LO 5.2] Laterality is indicated by the code with a specific number in the _____ or _____ position.
   a. Fifth, seventh
   b. Fourth, fifth
   c. Sixth, seventh
   d. Fifth, sixth

7. [LO 5.3] The tabular list is divided into _____.
   a. 17 chapters
   b. 21 chapters
   c. 17 plus E-codes
   d. 19 chapters

8. [LO 5.3] Symptoms, signs, and abnormal clinical and laboratory findings, not elsewhere classified, are found in category _____.
   a. R00–R99
   b. Z00–Z99
   c. Q00–Q99
   d. S00–T88

9. [LO 5.3] Diabetes mellitus would be found in Chapter _____.
   a. 5
   b. 8
   c. 4
   d. 19

10. [LO 5.4] When a code of less than six characters requires the use of a seventh character, you _____.
    a. Use 0
    b. Use z
    c. Use x
    d. Leave it blank

11. [LO 5.5] ICD-10-PCS is divided into _____ sections.
    a. 15
    b. 16
    c. 17
    d. 19

12. [LO 5.5] ICD-10-PCS is used to report services for _____.
    a. Outpatient facility procedures
    b. Office procedures only
    c. Inpatient hospital procedures
    d. None of the above

13. [LO 5.4] Categories always begin with a _____.
    a. Number
    b. Letter
    c. Number or letter
    d. Letter or number

14. [LO 5.1] GEM stands for _____.
    a. General equivalence marketing
    b. General equivalence motors
    c. Generally equivalence modifiers
    d. General equivalence mapping

15. [LO 5.1] ICD-10-PCS sections include all the following but _____.
   a. Medical and surgical
   b. Diagnoses
   c. Mental health
   d. Substance abuse treatment

16. [LO 5.4] Chronic tonsillitis and hypertrophy of the tonsils are reported by code(s) _____.
   a. J35.0, J35.1
   b. J35.01
   c. J35.1, J35.0
   d. J35.03

17. [LO 5.4] What code would you report for a pathological fracture of the left femur due to neoplastic disease?
   a. M84.552A, D49.2
   b. M84.529, D49.2
   c. M84.529
   d. M84.529A, D49.2

18. [LO 5.4] COPD with chronic bronchitis and emphysema is reported by code _____.
   a. J44.9
   b. J44.0, J42
   c. J18.9, E86.0
   d. J42

19. [LO 5.4] Dermatitis due to poison ivy is reported by code _____.
   a. L23
   b. L23.7
   c. L23.6
   d. L23.81

20. [LO 5.4] Martha has a diagnosis of non-Hodgkin lymphoma. What code is used to report Martha's diagnosis?
   a. C85.96
   b. C85.99
   c. C85.90
   d. C85.96

21. [LO 5.4] Febrile seizure is reported by code _____.
   a. R56.00
   b. R55
   c. P91
   d. R57.8

22. [LO 5.4] Angelika sustained a stress fracture. What is the code for her second doctor visit with regard to this injury?
   a. M84.31
   b. M84.371D
   c. M84.30xD
   d. M84.30xA

23. [LO 5.4] Alpers disease is reported using code _____.
   a. G31
   b. G31.84
   c. G31.81
   d. G31.9

24. [LO 5.4] Which code is used for the diagnosis of infantile autism?
   a. F84.5
   b. F84.0

**c.** F84.9

**d.** F84

**25.** [LO 5.4] A patient was diagnosed with left eye ghost vessels. This was reported using code _____.

   **a.** H16.412

   **b.** H16.419

   **c.** H16.41

   **d.** H16.399

## Applying Your Skills

Assign proper ICD-10-CM codes for the following diagnoses.

**1.** Follicular lichen planus. _____

**2.** Dorsal spina bifida with hydrocephalus. _____

**3.** General physical deterioration. _____

**4.** An HIV-positive pregnant woman in her first trimester. _____

**5.** Laceration of the scalp without foreign bodies present. _____

**6.** Carcinoma of the breast, 10 years ago, no evidence of recurrence. _____

**7.** Congenital bowing of left femur. _____

**8.** Typhoid arthritis. _____

**9.** Hypertension. _____

**10.** Adrenocortical crisis. _____

**11.** Congestive heart failure. _____

**12.** Diet-controlled gestational diabetes. _____

**13.** Gout. _____

**14.** Iron deficiency anemia. _____

**15.** Cancer of the floor of the mouth. _____

## Case Studies

For each of the following scenarios, assign the appropriate ICD-10-CM code(s).

**1.** [LO 5.4] A 27-year-old male comes to the office with a cough, fever, and six days of pronounced fatigue. He has taken Tylenol with no relief, and he has not had nausea or vomiting. His temperature is normal at 98.7; his BP 125/70; skin is normal; HEENT is normal; he is showing some redness in his throat; and all other areas are normal. Assessment is viral infection, so no antibiotics are to be given. _____

**2.** [LO 5.4] Alison is seen today to receive her second chemotherapy treatment for the diagnosis of acute lymphoid leukemia. Exam is normal, temperature 97.5, and BP 115/75. Chemotherapy was administered, and the patient tolerated the procedure well. _____

**3.** [LO .5.4] Quinn comes in with stomach cramping, vomiting, and diarrhea. Yesterday she had a chicken salad. Three hours later these symptoms began and have continued through the night. She is diagnosed with gastroenteritis, salmonella, abdominal cramping, vomiting, and diarrhea. _____

**4.** [LO 5.4] A 25-year-old man comes to the clinic today with known chronic hepatitis resulting from hepatitis B. He is suffering from delirium due to his chronic alcohol dependence. _____

**5.** [LO 5.4] A 50-year-old woman comes to the clinic today complaining of severe midepigastric pain with vomiting of bile. She had a CT scan yesterday, which confirmed the diagnosis of severe onset of inflammation of the gallbladder. She will be sent to Dr. Hoffman's for surgical evaluation. _____

**6.** [LO 5.4] Dorothy presents with a red swollen area on her right hip. After exam it is diagnosed that the patient has a sebaceous cyst. _____

7. [LO 5.4] A patient visits a clinic for evaluation of his third-degree burns of his left hand, 2 percent. Patient was seen five days ago for initial treatment. _____

8. [LO 5.4] An 18-year-old female visits her physician complaining of right flank pain. She hasn't noticed any fever or other discomforts. Her blood pressure is good at 110/70, temperature 98.5. UA was run, and the patient was found to have urinary tract infection. The patient was given antibiotics and educated on the need to complete the prescription even if she feels better. _____

9. [LO 5.4] Jennifer visits the hospital in her 38th week of pregnancy with labor pains. She was hooked up to the monitor, and a vaginal exam was completed to see how far she was dilated. It was determined after three hours that Jennifer was having false labor, and she was sent home. _____

10. [LO 5.4] Jacqui comes to the office today with acute abdominal pain. After a complete examination of the patient and a diagnostic x-ray film, it is determined that Jacqui has an acute small bowel obstruction. She is sent to the surgeon for evaluation and surgery. _____

## Thinking It Through

Using your critical-thinking skills, answer the following questions.

1. [LO 5.2] Explain why the physician needs to know a patient's family medical history. Under what circumstances would you code family history for a patient?

_____

_____

_____

_____

2. [LO 5.2] Explain the coding rules when a patient was born with a congenital malformation (such as a cleft palate) and has it corrected at some point in the patient's life.

_____

_____

_____

_____

3. [LO 5.2] Describe the coding rules as they apply to a patient who has asymptomatic HIV versus a patient who has a positive HIV test and is being treated for a HIV-related illness.

_____

_____

_____

_____

4. [LO 5.1] List two advantages of the implementation of ICD-10-CM in the United States.

_____

_____

_____

_____

5. [LO 5.1] Why is general equivalence mapping (GEM) not 100 percent accurate from ICD-9-CM to ICD-10-CM?

_____

_____

_____

_____

# 6

# INTRODUCTION TO CPT

## Learning Outcomes

*After completing this chapter, students should be able to:*

**6.1** Explain the structure of the CPT manual.

**6.2** Identify the information contained within each code section.

**6.3** Describe the functions of the index, appendixes, and additional information in the CPT manual.

**6.4** Describe the uses of Category II CPT codes.

**6.5** Differentiate the uses of Category III codes from those of Category I and Category II codes.

## Introduction

In addition to reporting patients' diagnoses and the reasons for medical encounters, coders must also report professional services using the Current Procedural Terminology (CPT) coding system. Learning how to code with CPT, just like ICD-9-CM, requires familiarity with the structure of the CPT manual. Coders must also be aware of general guidance on the use of the manual, differences between Category I, Category II, and Category III codes; meanings of symbols attached to some CPT codes; and general instructions on how to determine the correct code to report procedures and services described by these codes.

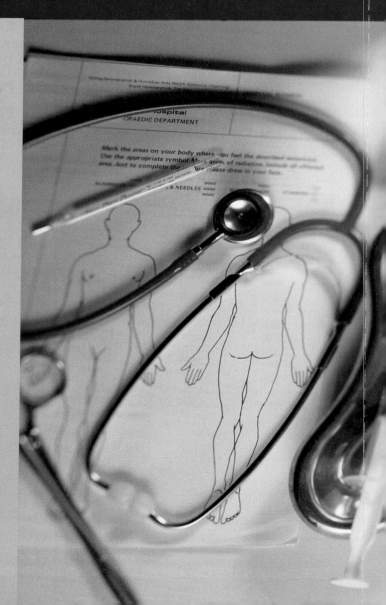

# Key Terms

Define each of the following key terms in the space provided.

1. [LO 6.1] CPT manual _____

_____

2. [LO 6.1, 6.5] Category I _____

_____

3. [LO 6.1, 6.5] Category III _____

_____

4. [LO 6.2] Code section _____

_____

5. [LO 6.5] Unlisted procedure _____

_____

6. [LO 6.1] Guidelines _____

_____

7. [LO 6.2] Symbols _____

_____

8. [LO 6.3] Add-on code _____

_____

9. [LO 6.2] Parent code _____

_____

10. [LO 6.3] Modifier 51 exempt _____

_____

11. [LO 6.2] Parenthetical note _____

_____

12. [LO 6.2] Modifier _____

_____

13. [LO 6.2] Separate procedure _____

_____

14. [LO 6.3] Index _____

_____

15. [LO 6.3] Appendix _____

_____

16. [LO 6.3] Main term _____

_____

17. [LO 6.3] Modifying term _____

_____

18. [LO 6.3] Place of service _____

_____

19. [LO 6.4] Performance measures _____

_____

**20.** [LO 6.4] Performance measurement exclusion modifier _____

_____

**21.** [LO 6.5] Emerging technology _____

_____

## Exam Review

Select the letter that best describes the statement or answers the question.

**1.** [LO 6.1] How many categories of codes are included in the CPT manual?

   **a.** 14

   **b.** 3

   **c.** 8

   **d.** 24

**2.** [LO 6.1] Which of the following categories describe services that are generally acceptable in the current practice of medicine?

   **a.** Category II

   **b.** Categories I and II

   **c.** Category IV

   **d.** Category I

**3.** [LO 6.1] Category I codes can be identified by which of the following?

   **a.** Five-digit code

   **b.** Up to five-digit code

   **c.** Alphanumeric code

   **d.** Two-digit code

**4.** [LO 6.1] Where would you locate a Category I code within the CPT manual?

   **a.** Pathology and laboratory

   **b.** Evaluation and management

   **c.** Surgery and anesthesia

   **d.** All of the above

**5.** [LO 6.1] Which of the following is true about Category I codes?

   **a.** Category I codes are always reimbursable.

   **b.** Category I codes are not always reimbursable.

   **c.** Category I codes are used to report performance measures.

   **d.** Category I codes are temporary codes.

**6.** [LO 6.1] Which of the following is used primarily for coding performance measures?

   **a.** Category III codes

   **b.** Category II codes

   **c.** Category I codes

   **d.** All of the above

**7.** [LO 6.1] For which of the following are Category II codes used?

   **a.** For reimbursement

   **b.** To designate emerging technologies

   **c.** To document the quality of services provided

   **d.** To increase the documentation

**8.** [LO 6.1] Which of the following can be said about Category II codes?

   **a.** They help document the extent to which services are provided in terms of number of providers.

   **b.** They help document trends of care in certain geographic regions.

    **c.** They contain four numeric digits followed by the letter *F*.

    **d.** All of the above.

**9.** [LO 6.1] How are Category II codes most useful?

    **a.** They reduce the manual efforts necessary to document services provided.

    **b.** They expedite the medical chart review process.

    **c.** They are used to determine if a code will eventually be included as a Category I code.

    **d.** Both (*a*) and (*b*).

**10.** [LO 6.1] Which of the following is true regarding Category III codes?

    **a.** Category III codes contain four numeric digits followed by the letter *T*.

    **b.** Category III codes document services to a patient population under care.

    **c.** Category III codes are permanent codes that document services.

    **d.** Category III codes are revised annually.

**11.** [LO 6.1] Which of the following can be said about Category I codes?

    **a.** They are mostly placed within numerical order within the CPT manual.

    **b.** They are organized by code sections according to the types of procedures.

    **c.** Category I codes include evaluation and management codes.

    **d.** All of the above.

**12.** [LO 6.1] To which of the three categories of codes do anesthesia, surgery, radiology, and medicine belong?

    **a.** Category III codes

    **b.** Category II codes

    **c.** Category I codes

    **d.** Category I and III codes

**13.** [LO 6.1] Which of the following is true about coding for the services that providers perform?

    **a.** Internal medicine physicians must only code from the Medicine Section of the CPT manual.

    **b.** For reporting purposes, coders must always use a Category II code along with other CPT codes.

    **c.** Providers can report codes from any and all sections of the CPT manual despite their medical specialty.

    **d.** Category II and III codes are not optional. They must be coded.

**14.** [LO 6.1] How many sections are located in Category I of the CPT manual?

    **a.** 14

    **b.** 5

    **c.** 6

    **d.** 10

**15.** [LO 6.1] Where are coding guidelines found within the CPT manual, and how are they best utilized?

    **a.** In the inside front cover of the manual; guidelines are used to report time spent performing services.

    **b.** In the appendix; they do not need to be used because the electronic billing systems and/or online coding information are adequate for coding purposes.

    **c.** At the end of each section; utilized by professors and health information technology personnel only.

    **d.** At the beginning of each section or category; read for understanding and specific coding instruction before coding.

**16.** [LO 6.2] Some sections of CPT codes consist of a main code with one or more indented codes following the main code. The indented codes share part of the definitions with the main code. Which of the following represents indented codes as they appear in the CPT manual?

    **a.** 61680    Surgery of intracranial arteriovenous malformation; supratentorial, simple;

          61682    Surgery of intracranial arteriovenous malformation; supratentorial, complex

    **b.** 61680    Surgery of intracranial arteriovenous malformation; supratentorial, simple

          61682       supratentorial, complex

          61684       infratentorial, simple

          61686       infratentorial, complex

    **c.** 27560    Closed treatment of patellar dislocation; without anesthesia

          27562       requiring anesthesia

    **d.** Both (*b*) and (*c*) are examples of main and indented codes in the CPT manual.

**17.** [LO 6.2] Which of the following symbols indicates a new procedure?

    **a.** ●

    **b.** ⊘

    **c.** ◉

    **d.** ▶ ◀

**18.** [LO 6.2] Which of the following symbols designates a code for vaccination pending approval from the Food and Drug Administration (FDA) listed in Appendix K?

    **a.** #

    **b.** ✚

    **c.** ⁄

    **d.** ▲

**19.** [LO 6.2] Which of the following is an add-on code that cannot be reported alone?

    **a.** ◉ 45330

    **b.** # 23071

    **c.** ▲ 22900

    **d.** ✚ 22614

**20.** [LO 6.1, 6.3] A patient suffers from obesity secondary to hypothyroidism and osteoarthritis, which limits his ability to exercise. The osteoarthritis (OA) is assessed, including the symptoms and functional status, and anti-inflammatory medication is prescribed. Which Category II code(s) would you report?

    **a.** 0005F

    **b.** 0005F and 1006F

    **c.** 1006F and 1007F

    **d.** 0521F

**21.** [LO 6.2] Which of the following is a "separate procedure" that should not be reported in addition to a code for the "total procedure"?

    **a.** 45380

    **b.** 57505

    **c.** 47460

    **d.** Both (*a*) and (*c*)

**22.** [LO 6.2] Parenthetical notes commonly direct the coder in the correct usage of the code(s) and may prohibit the use of certain code combinations. Which of the following is a code or group of codes that include a parenthetical note that provides specific instructions unique to those codes?

    **a.** 11010, 11011, 11012

    **b.** 64479–64495

    **c.** 43800

    **d.** All of the above

**23.** [LO 6.2] Which of the following coding examples may contain directions and/or instructions within parentheses?

    **a.** Add-on code 49905 Omental flap, intra-abdominal

    **b.** 20612 Aspiration and/or injection of ganglion cysts(s) any location

    **c.** Procedures that do not meet criteria for use of the code based upon requirements for the use of image guidance and must be reported with other codes

    **d.** All of the above

**24.** [LO 6.3] The CPT manual's index is organized alphabetically by main terms, including _____.

    **a.** A *procedure or service* (e.g., 49320 Diagnostic abdominal laparoscopy, 49321–49327 Surgical abdominal laparoscopy)

    **b.** A *condition* such as an abscess (e.g., 49040–49041 Abdominal abscess)

    **c.** An *organ or other anatomic site* such as in an Arthrocentesis of the elbow, 20605

    **d.** All of the above

**25.** [LO 6.2] When determining which code(s) to select for a certain procedure, coders should consider how certain terms may modify the nature and extent of the procedure performed. Which series of codes and/or range of codes describe a modification of the main procedure?

   **a.** 61332, 67400, 67450 Orbit Exploration (transcranial approach) with biopsy; Orbitotomy without bone flap (frontal or transconjunctival approach); for exploration, with or without biopsy; and Orbital exploration with or without biopsy.

   **b.** 23480–23485 Osteotomy, clavicle, with or without internal fixation; with bone graft for nonunion or malunion (includes obtaining graft and/or necessary fixation)

   **c.** 43752 Orogastric tube placement

   **d.** Both (a) and (b)

**26.** [LO 6.2] Which of the following codes would be reported for an otherwise healthy patient who had undergone laparoscopic surgery to rule out endometrioses.

   **a.** 49320 Diagnostic abdominal laparoscopy

   **b.** 00840 Anesthesia for intraperitoneal procedures in lower abdomen including laparoscopy; not otherwise specified

   **c.** Physical status modifier P1

   **d.** All of the above

**27.** [LO 6.1] A patient with a thyroid disease and secondary parathyroid disease has a low vitamin D level and is at risk for developing osteopenia and osteoporosis. The patient sees her primary care physician for complaints of back pain and right hip pain. X-rays and a bone density study of one or more sites of the axial skeleton are performed. The code for the bone density study is 77080. In what code category and section is this procedure found?

   **a.** Category III Medicine Section

   **b.** Category II and III Radiology Section

   **c.** Category I Radiology Section

   **d.** Category I Medicine Section

**28.** [LO6.4] Which of the following codes provides information related to patient safety?

   **a.** 4011F

   **b.** 27328

   **c.** 6015F

   **d.** 99213

**29.** [LO 6.3] Which of the following codes cannot be reported with modifier 63?

   **a.** 44127

   **b.** 33737

   **c.** 44120

   **d.** 33779

**30.** [LO 6.3] A 50-year-old man with acute chest pain and EKG changes consistent with an acute inferior myocardial infarction is seen in the hospital for the initial evaluation and management. Which of the following E/M codes might include a clinical example that is similar to the above scenario in Appendix C?

   **a.** 99223

   **b.** 99213

   **c.** 99233

   **d.** 99251

## Navigating the CPT Manual

Using your CPT manual, answer each of the following questions.

   **1.** [LO 6.3] A patient has metastatic adenocarcinoma and is under hospice care at home for end-of-life comfort. Where will you find a place of service code for this home care within the CPT manual?

**2.** [LO 6.1] A patient suffers a stroke and requires nasogastric tube placement in order to receive adequate nutrition. In which category and series of codes would the code for the tube placement be found?

_____

**3.** [LO 6.2, 6.3] A patient is seen on the same day during the same encounter for a secondary procedure that is significantly separate and identifiable from the primary procedure. In which appendix of the CPT manual will you find modifiers that may be added to procedural codes to indicate this scenario?

_____

**4.** [LO 6.1] A patient with a 20-year history of hypothyroidism develops a lump on the thyroid for which a fine needle biopsy is performed to determine if cancer is present or if the tumor is a benign goiter. In which category and section would the code for the fine needle biopsy be found?

_____

**5.** [LO 6.1] A 53-year-old male with a history of atherosclerotic heart disease presents to the emergency room with complaints of new onset of leg pain and a feeling that one leg is cooler to the touch than the other. It is determined that the patient has a femoral artery embolism for which a femoral artery embolectomy is performed. In which category and section would the code for the embolectomy be found?

_____

**6.** [LO 6.1, 6.3] A patient undergoes placement of a visceral extension prosthesis for endovascular repair of an abdominal aortic aneurysm involving visceral. This is described by CPT add-on code 0079T. In which appendix will you find the add-on code 0079T?

_____

**7.** [LO 6.3] Some codes are out of sequence within the CPT manual because they are better categorized with other procedures and no code numbers were available in that other section to classify the procedure. Where is a quick reference of these out-of-sequence codes found within the CPT manual? What symbol identifies these codes?

_____

**8.** [LO 6.1, 6.4] A patient is seen in the emergency room for irritability and depression. She is discharged with a referral to see a psychologist. In which code category and code section of the CPT manual would you find a code for the psychological counseling?

_____

**9.** [LO 6.1, 6.3] Some vaccine products have been assigned a CPT code in anticipation of future Food and Drug Administration (FDA) approval. Where might the coder find these codes within the CPT manual? What symbol identifies these codes?

_____

**10.** [LO 6.1] A patient has a postoperative abscess which requires drainage. In which code category and code section of the CPT manual would you expect to find the code that describes drainage of a postoperative abscess?

_____

**11.** [LO 6.3] A physician performs "an initial office visit for a patient with disseminated lupus erythematosus with kidney disease, edema, purpura, cardiac symptoms, and scarring lesions of the extremities." In which code category and section would a code describing this service likely be found in the CPT manual?

_____

**12.** [LO 6.3] A student studying to be a medical assistant is required to have an immunization record on file before she can begin her externship. She chooses to receive the hepatitis B vaccination. In which code category and section of the CPT manual is a code describing vaccinations found?

_____

**13.** [LO 6.1] It is suspected that a patient has sustained a systemic infection that has rendered the thyroid gland ineffective. A physician orders a total triiodothyronine test. In which category and section would the code for the thyroid test be found?

_____

**14.** [LO 6.3] A patient is admitted to the hospital for shortness of breath. Her physician sees her in the hospital during that time. In which code category and section of the CPT code manual will you find the CPT codes to describe the physician services provided to a hospitalized patient?

_____

**15.** [LO 6.1] A patient with non-Hodgkin lymphoma suffers a ruptured spleen requiring emergency surgical excision. In which code category and section is a code describing this surgical procedure likely to be found in the CPT manual?

_____

## Case Studies

For each of the following scenarios, identify where the appropriate CPT code(s) would be located, and answer the questions related to each case.

**1.** [LO 6.1, 6.2] A 36-year-old male is admitted to the hospital with breathlessness and cough. He has a history of being overweight, smoking and takes a beta-blocker for his hypertension. He works in commercial real estate and has had routine exposure to old industrial facilities with asbestos. Upon further evaluation, it is discovered that the patient has developed pulmonary edema for which a pneumocentesis is required to drain the fluid from his lungs. In which code category and section would the code describing the pneumocentesis be found?

_____

**2.** [LO 6.3] A physician's office is preparing for an audit by Medicare. While reviewing old claims, a billing manager and her staff discover they had reported some procedures with older codes that had been deleted from the CPT manual. They want to report those procedures using valid codes. Where in the CPT manual might they find a list of deleted older codes and the new codes that should be used to report those services?

_____

**3.** [LO 6.1, 6.2, 6.3] A 35-year-old patient with a history of multiple sclerosis, an autoimmune disease that affects the brain and spinal cord, is admitted to the hospital with complaints of decreased ability to move her arms, numbness in her legs, and loss of balance. The patient undergoes a nerve conduction test whereby electrodes are placed directly over the specific nerves to be tested. The medical record documentation specifies the following nerves to be tested: (a) musculo-cutaneous motor nerve to the biceps brachii and (b) femoral motor nerve to the vastus lateralis. Where in the CPT manual can the coder find a list of electrodiagnostic tests of sensory, motor, and mixed nerves?

_____

**4.** [LO 6.1, 6.4] A 36-year-old man was building a tree house for his young children when he fell from the tree and sustained a spinal cord injury of the neck. He was rendered a quadriplegic and will be ventilator-dependent for the remainder of his life. He and his wife are deciding what care he wants to receive in the future. They discuss "do not resuscitate" (DNR) orders with the physician. Where in the CPT manual would the physician find codes to document these advanced care planning discussion?

_____

**5.** [LO 6.1, 6.4] A patient presents to her primary care physician with complaints of unusual psychic events, such as seeing auras around people and objects and ocular migraines. She also believes she can tell the future. A psychiatric diagnosis is ruled out, and the patient is referred to a neurologist who conducts a variety of neurological tests including a MRI. The physician documents temporal lobe epilepsy (TLE) in the patient's chart. The patient is placed on anticonvulsant medication. The medical record further notes that the physician monitored the therapeutic levels of her medications. In which category and section of the CPT manual would you find a code for reporting the documentation of therapeutic monitoring of an anticonvulsant medication that has been ordered or performed?

_____

**6.** [LO 6.1, 6.4] A 32-year-old woman is seen by her gynecologist because she has been emotionally labile with aggression and depressive tendencies. TSH, estrogen, progesterone, testosterone, and other hormone levels are checked. Premenstrual dysphoric disorder (PMDD) and other hormone imbalances are ruled out. A psychiatrist performs a mental status assessment. In which code category and section would the code for this assessment be found?

_____

**7.** [LO 6.1, 6.4] A patient diagnosed with diabetes and obesity is placed on a protein sparing modified diet consisting of low carbohydrates. After three weeks of obesity intervention with the hopes of improving the diabetic condition, the patient is admitted to the emergency room after experiencing weakness, fatigue, increased thirst and urination, and vomiting. The patient is found to be in ketoacidosis and mildly dehydrated. IV fluids are administered. In which code category and section of the CPT manual would codes describing treatment in the emergency room be found?

_____

**8.** [LO 6.1, 6.4] A 50-year-old male has had episodes of excruciating chest pain that radiates into his jaws for the past 10 years. His EKG and laboratory tests are normal, indicating that he has not had a myocardial infarction. The treating physician believes the patient is suffering from gastroesophageal reflux disease (GERD), but refers the patient to a pulmonologist for an evaluation to rule out pulmonary disease as a cause of the chest pain. The pulmonologist evaluates the patient, performs screening tests of his pulmonary function, and determines that the patient does not have chronic obstructive pulmonary disease (COPD). In which code category would a code documenting that the physician performed an evaluation of pulmonary function likely be found?

_____

**9.** [LO 6.1, 6.4] A 26-year-old female experiences tunnel vision, shortness of breath, tachycardia, and extreme anxiety while driving. The patient is hyperventilating when she presents to the emergency room for evaluation. The patient has a full workup, which includes an electrocardiogram (EKG). In which category and section would a code describing the EKG be found? In which code category would a code documenting that the physician performed the EKG be found?

_____

_____

**10.** [LO 6.1, 6.4] A patient presents to emergency psychiatric services with her husband because he is concerned that his wife is not getting enough sleep. The wife is up all hours of the night after sniffing toluene. She claims to talk with skeletons coming out of her coffee table. The constant chatter is preventing her husband from getting the sleep he needs. A psychological evaluation, which includes a history, mental status exam, and disposition, is obtained. The medical record states that the patient is referred for psychotherapy to treat her diagnoses of drug addiction and mental illness. In which category and section would the code documenting the psychiatric referral be found?

_____

**11.** [LO 6.1, 6.5] A 48-year-old male with a previous history of sinus surgery is seen because his wife notices that he has episodes during sleep when his breathing stops for a prolonged period of time. The physician suspects that the patient has sleep apnea. The patient undergoes a sleep study to evaluate the extent of this problem. The physician orders this test using a new technology that the physician believes will provide more information than the usual sleep study In which code category might the code for this new sleep study be found?

_____

**12.** [LO 6.1, 6.5] A 35-year-old patient has been feeling malaise and fatigue for several weeks. She also complains of episodic tachycardia. After completing a series of lab tests, her primary care physician refers her to a hematologist for further evaluation. The hematologist orders further laboratory tests and bone marrow biopsy. What code category are codes describing these services likely to be found? Identify as many sections of CPT codes as you can that might contain codes describing services and procedures provided to this patient.

_____

_____

**13.** [LO 6.3] During arterial catheterization procedures, the physician threads a catheter through the aorta into major arteries, sometimes referred to as first-order vessels. The physician may continue to thread the catheter into smaller arteries, referred to as second-order and third-order vessels. Where in the CPT manual might a coder find a list of vessels that are considered first-order, second-order, and third-order vessels, which are collectively referred to as vascular families?

_____

**14.** [LO 6.1, 6.3] A 36-year-old male patient sees his pulmonologist because he is coughing up blood (hemoptysis). The pulmonologist performs a pneumonostomy, with percutaneous drainage of an abscess secondary to pneumonia. Radiological supervision and interpretation were required for fluoroscopic guidance. In which code category and section would the codes describing the pneumostomy and radiological supervision and guidance be found?

_____

**15.** [LO 6.3] Nuclear cardiology and radioactive radiological procedures aid in the diagnosis of cardiology conditions. These procedures involve the injection of radioactive substances into the blood system and taking special images of the heart to identify possible conditions involving the coronary arteries. In which category and section of the CPT manual would the codes for these radiological procedures be found?

_____

## Thinking It Through

Using your critical-thinking skills, answer the questions below.

**1.** [LO 6.2, 6.3] A patient's physician suspects she may have familial dysautonomia, which is a genetic disorder found in the Ashkenazi population. Cytogenetic studies are ordered to test for oncologic or inherited disorders. Genetic testing modifiers are reported with molecular laboratory procedures related to genetic testing. Where might you find genetic testing modifiers in the CPT manual? What do the guidelines say about how these codes are reported?

_____

_____

_____

**2.** [LO 6.1] Assume a patient has a condition, such as an infection, that requires an incision and drainage of the elbow. Identify the code category where the appropriate code is likely to be located. Assuming this is likely to be performed in a hospital, discuss the types of services that are usually reported for this type of procedure (hint: think of different medical providers that may provide services during a hospital stay for this procedure).

_____

_____

_____

**3.** [LO 6.2] Coders should be aware of procedures that are separate from or integral to one another. Identify some indicators in the CPT manual that one procedure is usually integral to another procedure. Describe the circumstances that might support reporting those procedures as separate or distinct procedures.

_____

_____

_____

**4.** [LO 6.1, 6.2] A marathon runner has a chief complaint of knee pain for over one month and is unable to run in any more marathons due to excruciating knee pain. The orthopedic surgeon decides to do a diagnostic arthroscopy to determine if further surgery is warranted. The procedure is performed under local anesthesia until a complication arises requiring general anesthesia. Identify the code category to describe this procedure. How would you identify the correct code using general information found in the CPT manual?

_____

_____

_____

**5.** [LO 6.1] Chronic glomerulonephritis has damaged a patient's right kidney. A surgeon performs a laparoscopic nephrectomy. The adrenal gland, which sits on top of the kidney, also needs to be removed. Of the six sections in Category I of the CPT manual, identify the sections that likely contain codes to describe these procedures.

_____

_____

_____

_____

# MODIFIERS

## Learning Outcomes

*After completing this chapter, students should be able to:*

**7.1** Explain the functions and uses of modifiers.

**7.2** Discuss modifiers to indicate services provided during a procedure's global period.

**7.3** Use modifiers to report components of procedures or services.

**7.4** Explain bilateral, multiple, repeat, or additional procedures performed on the same date of service.

**7.5** Cite appropriate modifiers to identify individuals who assist the primary provider during procedures.

**7.6** Discuss circumstances where the amount of work necessary to perform the service differs significantly from the amount typically necessary.

**7.7** Define modifiers describing mandatory services, physical status, and genetic tests.

**7.8** Define HCPCS modifiers to primary codes.

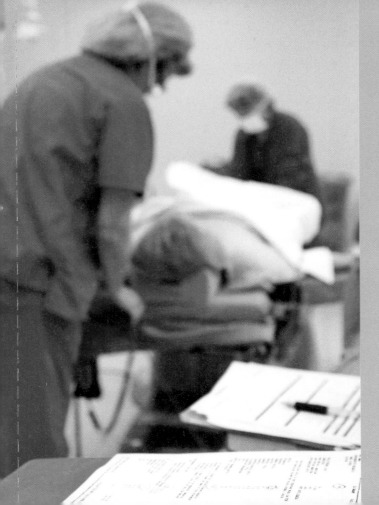

## Introduction

Modifiers are two-digit alphanumeric characters that are added to CPT or HCPCS codes to provide additional information. CPT and HCPCS codes do not always fully describe services provided with as much detail as is available in the medical record. Coders must understand how to use modifiers correctly to convey that additional information. It is critical to know as much about selecting modifiers as about selecting codes.

There are two major types of modifiers: payment modifiers and informational modifiers. *Payment modifiers* usually affect the amount of the payment for services described by the codes to which the modifiers are attached. *Informational modifiers,* on the other hand, do not typically affect payments, but may do so.

## Key Terms

Fill in each blank with the key term that best completes the sentence.

1. [LO 7.1] The _____ codes are used to report physician services in the office/outpatient setting, inpatient facility, emergency department, nursing homes, and domiciliary care.

2. [LO 7.2] The _____ modifier reports the use of equipment and supplies for some services when the use of the equipment is reported separately from the professional expertise involved in providing the service.

3. [LO 7.4] _____ are when the surgeon performs an additional procedure that is not considered a bundled component of the primary procedure.

4. [LO 7.5] When a resident physician functions as an aide to the surgeon during the performance of surgical procedures, the resident is acting as a(n) _____.

5. [LO 7.3] When a radiologist provides expertise to review an x-ray that was produced on equipment owned by another entity, the service is reported with the _____ modifier.

6. [LO 7.5] When two surgeons work together to perform different parts of the procedure, the surgeons would use the _____ modifier to report their services.

7. [LO 7.4] The patient had a total hip replacement on both the right and left during the same operative procedure. This is considered a(n) _____.

8. [LO 7.2] Each CPT procedure has a number of days assigned that are considered the _____, during which time many physician services are considered part of the underlying procedure.

9. [LO 7.1] When a surgeon plans a surgery to follow at some point in time after the first surgery, this is considered a(n) _____.

10. [LO 7.2] After evaluating a patient, a surgeon may make the _____, if the surgeon thinks surgical intervention is the preferred treatment option.

11. [LO 7.7] _____ modifiers designate the underlying health of the patient and are reported by anesthesiologists.

12. [LO 7.5] Transplant patients often have a(n) _____ because of the complexity of the procedures.

13. [LO 7.5] Surgeons who are still supervised by their attending physicians are referred to as _____.

14. [LO 7.8] Right and left side of the body, specific fingers, toes, eyelids, and certain coronary arteries are identified with _____.

## Exam Review

Select the letter that best describes the statement or answers the question.

1. [LO 7.1] Modifiers may be used to indicate which of the following type(s) of information?
   a. Bilateral procedures
   b. Canceled procedures
   c. Staged procedures
   d. All of the above

2. [LO 7.7] A patient's insurance company required a second opinion prior to surgery. The coder should use which modifier to report that service?
   a. 22
   b. 32
   c. 24
   d. 57

3. [LO 7.8] Modifier AA is an example of what type of modifier?
   a. HCPCS
   b. CPT

    **c.** ICD-9-CM

    **d.** None of the above

4. [LO 7.2] Modifier 25 is only added to codes reporting which of the following services?

    **a.** Inpatient services

    **b.** Nursing home services

    **c.** Office or outpatient services

    **d.** Evaluation and management services

5. [LO 7.2] Modifier 79 (unrelated procedure or service by the same physician during the postoperative period) is used for what type of services?

    **a.** Surgery

    **b.** E/M

    **c.** Anesthesia

    **d.** All of the above

6. [LO 7.2] A return to the operating room for an unplanned related procedure or service by the same physician during the postoperative period calls for which modifier?

    **a.** 77

    **b.** 78

    **c.** 79

    **d.** 76

7. [LO 7.4] Modifier 59 is used to indicate that _____.

    **a.** The patient was taken back to the operating room for a complication relating to the previous surgery

    **b.** A subsequent surgery was planned or staged

    **c.** A distinct and separate procedure was performed concurrently with another

    **d.** None of the above

8. [LO 7.8] When a patient is transported by ambulance, a modifier must be appended to the base transportation code to describe which of the following events?

    **a.** If the patient was ambulatory when picked up

    **b.** Whether a family member rode with the patient

    **c.** Where the patient was picked up and dropped off

    **d.** Whether the patient was stable during the transport

9. [LO 7.4] The modifier that indicates multiple procedures is:

    **a.** 25

    **b.** 32

    **c.** 59

    **d.** 51

10. [LO 7.6] What does modifier 63 describe?

    **a.** Procedure performed on infants less than 4 kg

    **b.** Procedure performed on infants less than 6 kg

    **c.** Procedure performed on infants more than 8 kg

    **d.** Procedure performed on critically ill patients

11. [LO 7.4] If a clinical lab needs to be repeated, it is reported with which modifier?

    **a.** 99

    **b.** 90

    **c.** 91

    **d.** 92

12. [LO 7.7] Modifiers P1–P6 are used to describe the patient's _____.

    **a.** Age

    **b.** Weight

**c.** Health status

**d.** Age and weight

13. [LO 7.8]  Which modifier is reported to indicate that a surgeon performed a procedure on the left ankle of a patient?

    **a.** 59

    **b.** RT

    **c.** F1

    **d.** LT

14. [LO 7.1]  Which of the following situations can be described by the use of a modifier?

    **a.** Only part of the service was performed.

    **b.** Multiple procedures were performed.

    **c.** The service was complicated and unusual.

    **d.** All of the above.

15. [LO 7.6]  Corrine is scheduled for a gallbladder removal. As the procedure begins, her blood pressure rises and the procedure is stopped. The decision is made to cancel the procedure. Which modifier would be appended to the surgical procedure?

    **a.** 74.

    **b.** 53.

    **c.** None (The procedure will not be billed.)

    **d.** Anesthesia is the only code that can be used.

16. [LO 7.1]  What is the "surgical care only" modifier?

    **a.** 57

    **b.** 32

    **c.** 66

    **d.** 54

17. [LO 7.7]  The physical status of a brain-dead patient whose organs are being removed for donor purposes is reported using modifier _____.

    **a.** P2

    **b.** P4

    **c.** P6

    **d.** P5

18. [LO 7.5]  If the surgical procedure requires surgeons of different specialties at the same operative session, which modifier would each surgeon use?

    **a.** 62

    **b.** 80

    **c.** 82

    **d.** 66

19. [LO 7.8]  James has multiple lacerations with tendon involvement on his right hand, which requires repair of the second digit, third digit, and fourth digit. Which modifiers would be appended to each procedure?

    **a.** E1, E2, E3

    **b.** FA, F5, F6

    **c.** F6, F7, F8

    **d.** F4, F6, F9

20. [LO 7.5]  When more than two physicians work together on a complicated procedure and each physician has a specific portion of the surgery to complete, they would add which modifier to the code that describes the procedures?

    **a.** 66

    **b.** 80

    **c.** 62

    **d.** 82

21. [LO 7.3] Theresa is sent to an imaging center for an MRI of her spine. The imaging center does not employ a radiologist to read the film, so a radiologist is called in. Which modifier does the imaging center add to the codes that describes its MRI service?

   **a.** 26
   **b.** None
   **c.** 51
   **d.** TC

22. [LO 7.4] Perry comes to outpatient surgery for an arthroscopic knee procedure involving a lateral meniscectomy and limited synovectomy of the medial compartment. Which modifier is added to the arthroscopic synovectomy code 29875?

   **a.** 51
   **b.** 52
   **c.** 59
   **d.** None, the procedure is unbilled.

23. [LO 7.2] Belinda returns to her physician's office for follow-up during the global period of a procedure to remove a ganglion cyst from her hand. While in the office, she complains of knee pain. Which modifier is used for the E/M services related to the knee?

   **a.** 24
   **b.** 25
   **c.** 78
   **d.** None of these

24. [LO .2] Modifier 24 should only be used with _____.

   **a.** E/M codes
   **b.** Pathology
   **c.** Radiology
   **d.** Surgical procedures

25. [LO 7.7] A patient is disabled with a back injury. The insurance company paying for his short-term disability requires him to see its company physician in order for benefits to continue. Which modifier will the physician's office append to the E/M code?

   **a.** 24
   **b.** 25
   **c.** 32
   **d.** No modifier needed

26. [LO 7.3] The portion of a test involving a professional interpretation only is reported with which modifier added to the code that describes the service?

   **a.** 22
   **b.** TC
   **c.** 26
   **d.** No modifier needed.

27. [LO 7.2] Mr. Taylor comes back to the outpatient department today for a planned second grafting procedure after a severe third-degree burn. The first procedure was performed 30 days ago and has a global period of 90 days. Which modifier is added to the surgery CPT codes?

   **a.** 22
   **b.** 57
   **c.** 58
   **d.** None—the patient is past the global period.

**28.** [LO 7.4]  Miss Leonard comes in for outpatient surgical rotator cuff repair. While the patient is under general anesthesia, the surgeon will also remove her ingrown toenails. Which modifier is appended to the codes for the toenail procedure?

    **a.** 51

    **b.** 22

    **c.** 59

    **d.** 52

**29.** [LO 7.5]  The patient has a closed treatment of the third and fourth metatarsal fractures with manipulation. Which modifier is appended to the second procedure?

    **a.** 59

    **b.** 51

    **c.** 52

    **d.** None

**30.** [LO 7.1]  Modifiers may affect the reimbursement by _____.

    **a.** Increasing the amount

    **b.** Decreasing the amount

    **c.** Modifiers do not affect reimbursement

    **d.** Both (*a*) and (*b*)

## Applying Your Skills

Identify the appropriate modifiers for each of the following situations.

**1.** [LO 7.3]  When coding the professional component of a procedure, use modifier _____.

**2.** [LO 7.4]  Johan had multiple procedures done during the same operative session. _____

**3.** [LO 7.4]  If the facility provides the x-ray but does not have a radiologist employed, the facility would use modifier _____ for its radiology code.

**4.** [LO 7.2]  When a related second procedure is performed during the postoperative period, modifier _____ would be appended.

**5.** [LO 7.8]  A surgeon performs a bunionectomy on the right great toe of a patient. Which modifier is added to the code that describes the procedure? _____

**6.** [LO 7.5]  When two surgeons work together as primary surgeons performing distinct parts of a procedure, each should report which modifier to the procedure code? _____

**7.** [LO 7.8]  The surgeon performs a therapeutic interventional procedure on the right coronary artery of a patient. Which modifier is added to the code? _____

**8.** [LO 7.4]  When clinical lab tests are repeated on the same day, which modifier would be appended? _____

**9.** [LO 7.4]  When a surgeon performs identical procedures on both the left and right knees, modifier _____ would be used.

**10.** [LO 7.8]  A surgeon performs a left eyelid blepharoplasty. Which modifier would be used with the CPT code? _____

**11.** [LO 7.6]  The patient has a surgical procedure done by Dr. Arlington. An anesthesiologist was not available so the surgeon administered the anesthesia in addition to performing the surgery. Which modifier will be appended to the code? _____

**12.** [LO 7.7]  The anesthesiologist reports that a patient has uncontrolled hypertension and is a brittle diabetic. Which modifier would be appended to the anesthesia code? _____

**13.** [LO 7.5]  Modifier _____ is used to indicate that an assistant surgeon provided services in a teaching hospital when a qualified resident surgeon was not available.

**14.** [LO 7.1]  The patient comes in for a postoperative office visit. The physician would use which modifier? _____

**15.** [LO 7.1] The patient comes to the office with a nondisplaced fracture of the arm. Due to the patient's mental status, the decision is made to take him to outpatient surgery and apply the cast under anesthesia, even though that is not usually necessary. Modifier _____ is added to the code.

## Case Studies

Read each case study and select the appropriate modifier to describe each case.

**1.** [LO 7.2] Sam presented to his physician complaining of a severe sore throat. The physician examined him and prescribed antibiotics. While performing the exam, the physician offered to remove a mole. The physician reports both procedures. Which modifier would be appended to the E/M visit for that day?

_____

**2.** [LO 7.7] Mrs. Parker fell while at her local supermarket and, as required, visited the company's physician to be sure she was all right. Which modifier would be appended to the E/M visit? _____

**3.** [LO 7.5] Dr. Roberts is performing a total knee replacement on his patient. His partner, Dr. Cooper, assists with the procedure. Which modifier would Dr. Cooper use to report her services? _____

**4.** [LO 7.2] Gary had a cataract removed from his right eye by Dr. Holmes. While Gary was still in his postoperative recovery period, Dr. Holmes opted to remove a cataract from his left eye as well. Which modifier would be appended to the second cataract removal? _____

**5.** [LO 7.2] A patient visits her physician for a follow-up exam after an appendectomy. The patient complains of a sore throat and earache. After examining the patient, the physician diagnoses sinusitis and otitis media. Which modifier will the physician add to the code that describes the E/M services? _____

**6.** [LO 7.6] Mrs. Watkins has a total hip replacement. Due to the patient's extreme morbid obesity, the procedure takes several hours longer than usual. The surgeon documents the difficulty he had accessing the hip and maneuvering the prosthesis. Which modifier would be appended to the procedure code? _____

**7.** [LO 7.6] The physician requests one view of the right elbow. Which modifier would be appended to 73070? _____

**8.** [LO 7.3] Dr. Yi performed a cataract surgery on his patient. Dr. Jones then provided the postoperative care following discharge. Which modifier would Dr. Jones use to document that she only provided postoperative care? _____

**9.** [LO 7.8] A surgeon performs surgery on her patient's left thumb. What would be the proper HCPCS modifier to add to the CPT procedure code? _____

**10.** [LO 7.2] Dr. McManis places a pacemaker in a patient before traveling out of town. While Dr. McManis is away, a complication forces his colleague, Dr. Romero, to repeat the procedure. Which modifier would be appended to the code reporting Dr. Romero's surgery? _____

## Thinking It Through

Using your critical-thinking skills, answer the following questions.

**1.** [LO 7.1, 7.8] Explain the two levels of modifiers within HCPCS. Who maintains these modifiers?

_____

_____

_____

_____

**2.** [LO 7.1]  In general terms, how can modifiers affect payment for procedures?

_____

_____

_____

_____

**3.** [LO 7.6]  When the physician adds modifier 22 to a procedure code, what type of information should she be prepared to provide if requested to do so?

_____

_____

_____

_____

**4.** [LO 7.2] A new patient visits a physician because of a painful knee. The physician completes the patient's history, physical exam, and medical decision making. After reviewing the case, the physician makes the decision to treat the patient's knee with a cortisone injection. Can the physician bill for the evaluation and management visit as well as the cortisone injection? If so, which modifier would be used?

_____

_____

_____

_____

**5.** [LO 7.8]  Describe the circumstances under which the GA modifier may be added to a code.

_____

_____

_____

_____

# EVALUATION AND MANAGEMENT SERVICES, PART I: STRUCTURE AND GUIDANCE

## Learning Outcomes

*After completing this chapter, students should be able to:*

**8.1** Explain the breakdown of E/M services into categories and subcategories.

**8.2** Define key terms related to E/M coding.

**8.3** Determine the level of various E/M codes based on primary and secondary components.

**8.4** Differentiate among the four types of histories.

**8.5** Contrast the four types of physical examinations.

**8.6** Differentiate among the four types of medical decision making.

**8.7** Explain how the key components determine the level of E/M services provided.

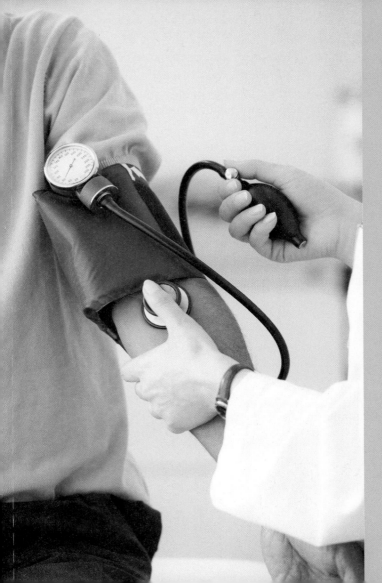

## Introduction

Evaluation and management (E/M) codes describe a wide range of physician services commonly associated with doctor visits, such as taking the patient's history, performing a physical examination, ordering and interpreting laboratory and radiological tests, determining the cause of the patient's condition, prescribing appropriate treatments, and monitoring the patient for changes in his or her condition. It is often more difficult to select the appropriate E/M code than to identify a procedure code.

Selecting the correct E/M code depends on multiple elements, each of which is made up of several levels. The level of each element must be determined to select the correct E/M code. This chapter describes each element, how to determine the level of those elements, and how the elements are used to determine the specific E/M code to describe the overall service.

# Key Terms

Fill in each blank with the key term that best completes the sentence.

1. [LO 8.1] A(n) _____ is a patient who has not been seen by the physician or group practice during the previous three years.

2. [LO 8.2] _____ describes discussion with a patient and/or family regarding aspects of the patient's medical situation.

3. [LO 8.4] A review of the patient's previous major illnesses, injuries, operations, hospitalizations, medications, allergies, immunizations, and dietary status is a(n) _____.

4. [LO 8.5] The _____ is the process by which a physician or other healthcare provider assesses a patient for the presence of or extent of an illness or injury.

5. [LO 8.1] History, physical examination, and medical decision making are _____ used to determine the E/M level.

6. [LO 8.1] The _____ is a chronological description of the development of the patient's current problem.

7. [LO 8.1] _____ cover a broad range of physician services commonly associated with "doctor visits."

8. [LO 8.1] A patient who has been seen by the physician or another physician of the same specialty in the group practice during the previous three years is called a(n) _____.

9. [LO 8.4] The _____ is a review of the medical history of family members that includes health status and cause of death.

10. [LO 8.2] The reason for an encounter with a physician, with or without a definitive diagnosis, is called the _____.

11. [LO 8.2] A complete _____ must include at least one specific item from the following history areas: past medical history, family history, and social history.

12. [LO 8.2] The _____ is a series of questions regarding body and organ systems designed to identify signs and symptoms.

13. [LO 8.6] Consideration of all available information—including history, exams, tests, imaging studies, and other information—to determine possible diagnoses and treatment options for the patient's condition is called _____.

14. [LO 8.2] The _____ is a review of the patient's nonmedical information, including current employment, occupational history, marital status, education, sexual history, and use of alcohol, tobacco, and drugs.

15. [LO 8.7] _____ is an explicit and variable component of most E/M services.

16. [LO 8.2] The _____ used to determine the E/M level are counseling, care coordination, and the nature of the presenting problem.

17. [LO 8.1] _____ occurs when two or more physicians provide care to the same patient on the same day.

18. [LO 8.1] Delivery of medical care to a critically ill or injured patient is _____.

19. [LO 8.1] A(n) _____ is a service provided by a physician when another physician requests an opinion or advice.

# Exam Review

Select the letter that best describes the statement or answers the question.

1. [LO 8.3] Which of the following is *not* a key component for determining an E/M level of service?
   a. Physical examination
   b. History
   c. Care coordination
   d. Medical decision making

2. [LO 8.4] How many body systems must be addressed and documented in a complete review of systems (ROS)?
   a. Two to nine
   b. Ten or more
   c. Eight or more
   d. All systems

3. [LO 8.1] What is the initial question the coder must ask when reporting E/M services?
   a. Where were the services provided?
   b. Is the patient a new patient?
   c. What is the patient's age?
   d. Is the visit an initial or subsequent visit?

4. [LO 8.6] A general multisystem exam is also called _____.
   a. A detailed exam
   b. An expanded problem-focused exam
   c. A physical exam
   d. A comprehensive exam

5. [LO 8.2] The chief complaint is _____.
   a. A review of the patient's present illness
   b. A brief statement that describes the reason for a transfer of care
   c. A brief statement that describes the reason the patient is seeing the physician
   d. The most important symptom

6. [LO 8.2] Education of a patient or patient's family regarding aspects of a medical situation is considered
   _____.
   a. Counseling
   b. Transfer of care
   c. Medical decision making
   d. Treatment compliance

7. [LO 8.2] A patient has a problem that runs a prescribed course or is short-lived. This is what type of presenting problem?
   a. Minimal
   b. Moderate severity
   c. Low severity
   d. Self-limited or minor

8. [LO 8.2] A review of a patient's use of alcohol, tobacco, or drugs is a component of _____.
   a. Family history
   b. Medical history
   c. Social history
   d. Review of systems

9. [LO 8.5] Which of the following is *not* a distinct body area recognized for E/M coding purposes?
   a. Skin
   b. Head and or/face
   c. Genitalia, groin, buttocks
   d. Neck

10. [LO 8.7] How many decision-making elements must meet or exceed the requirements to assign a type of decision-making complexity?
    a. All requirements
    b. One out of three
    c. Two out of three
    d. Either (*a*) or (*c*)

11. [LO 8.1] Which of the following categories of E/M codes are primarily determined by the location in which services were provided?

    **a.** Newborn services
    **b.** Emergency department services
    **c.** Consultations
    **d.** Either (*b*) or (*c*)

12. [LO 8.2] A patient who has been to the emergency department five times in two months and has been treated by the same physician on multiple occasions is a _____.

    **a.** New patient
    **b.** Hypochondriac
    **c.** Established patient
    **d.** Recurring patient

13. [LO 8.2] Concurrent care occurs when how many physicians provide care to the same patient on the same day?

    **a.** One
    **b.** Three or more
    **c.** Four or more
    **d.** Two or more

14. [LO 8.2] Severity, duration, modifying factors, and quality are all elements of the _____.

    **a.** History of present illness
    **b.** Review of systems
    **c.** Past medical history
    **d.** Either (*a*) or (*b*)

15. [LO 8.7] How many key components must meet or exceed the requirements of the selected level of E/M services for an initial inpatient consultation?

    **a.** Two out of three
    **b.** One plus two contributory components
    **c.** All three
    **d.** There are no requirements for a consultation

## Applying Your Skills

Read each question and provide the correct answer.

1. [LO 8.1] What three questions must be answered before dividing E/M services into subcategories?

    **a.** _____

    **b.** _____

    **c.** _____

2. [LO 8.6] When determining the type of medical decision making required, identify three factors that must be taken into consideration:

    **a.** _____

    **b.** _____

    **c.** _____

3. [LO 8.4] What are the five types of presenting problems associated with E/M coding?

    **a.** _____

    **b.** _____

    **c.** _____

    **d.** _____

    **e.** _____

**4.** [LO 8.7]  What factors must be considered when choosing the correct E/M code?

_____

_____

_____

**5.** [LO 8.5]  What is the main difference between a problem-focused physical exam and an expanded problem-focused physical exam?

_____

_____

_____

**6.** [LO 8.7]  Identify three of the major categories of E/M services.

a. _____

b. _____

c. _____

**7.** [LO 8.4]  What are the four types of history that are taken into account when coding?

a. _____

b. _____

c. _____

d. _____

**8.** [LO 8.3]  E/M codes have a set format that is more extensive than most other CPT codes. What are some of the components in the E/M code format?

_____

_____

**9.** [LO 8.6]  What are the four types of medical decision making?

a. _____

b. _____

c. _____

d. _____

**10.** [LO 8.3]  Of the seven components used to define the level of E/M services provided, _____ is/are variable.

**11.** [LO 8.6]  What requirements must be met for straightforward medical decision making?

_____

_____

_____

**12.** [LO 8.5]  When performing a general multisystem exam, how many of the organ systems must be examined?

_____

**13.** [LO 8.4]  Past history reviews the patient's _____.

**14.** [LO 8.6]  Aside from the amount of possible diagnoses, treatment options, and data, what is the difference between low-complexity medical decision making and moderate-complexity medical decision making?

_____

**15.** [LO 8.4]  A(n) _____ is a problem that usually runs a prescribed course and does not usually permanently change the patient's health status.

_____

**16.** [LO 8.6] High-complexity medical decision making must meet what requirements?

_____

_____

## Case Studies

Read each case study. Using your knowledge of the factors of E/M coding, answer the questions that follow each case.

**1.** [LO 8.6] Jake broke his arm falling from his tree house. His physician, Dr. King, refers him to an orthopedic surgeon whom Jake has seen within the last three years for other problems. The orthopedic surgeon performs an expanded problem-focused history and examination. The surgeon has to consider multiple diagnoses and treatment options, review a fair amount of data, and face a moderate risk of complications if Jake's growth plate is damaged. What level of medical decision making would this be classified as?

_____

_____

**2.** [LO 8.6] Mr. Takahari is rushed to the ER with a gunshot wound to the chest. The ER attending physician performs a comprehensive history and a comprehensive examination, and his medical decision making is of high complexity. Why would this be considered high complexity?

_____

_____

**3.** [LO 8.2] Nathan has been repeatedly hospitalized for heroin abuse and has entered a rehabilitation program. Once a week, a physician leads Nathan and a group of recovering addicts in a risk reduction intervention counseling session. Each session lasts approximately 60 minutes. Is this considered counseling for purposes of selecting the appropriate level of E/M code? Why or why not?

_____

_____

## Thinking It Through

Using your critical-thinking skills, answer the following questions.

**1.** [LO 8.4] Describe the four types of patient history and the elements that determine which type has been provided as part of an E/M service.

_____

_____

_____

_____

**2.** [LO 8.5] List the four types of physical examination and the factors that determine which type has been provided as part of an E/M service.

_____

_____

_____

_____

**3.** [LO 8.6]  Discuss the four types of medical decision making. What differentiates the factors from one another?

_____

_____

_____

_____

**4.** [LO 8.7]  Describe in general terms the types of E/M services requiring that three out of three factors meet or exceed the levels in the code descriptors and those only requiring that two out of three factors meet or exceed the levels in the code descriptors. How do coders know for certain how many are required?

_____

_____

_____

_____

**5.** [LO 8.7]  Describe the circumstances under which the key components do not determine the level of E/M services provided and the contributory components are used instead to determine those services.

_____

_____

_____

_____

## Learning Outcomes

*After completing this chapter, students should be able to:*

**9.1** Explain how differences between new and established patients affect E/M code selection in outpatient settings.

**9.2** Differentiate among various categories and subcategories of hospital services.

**9.3** Describe how consultation codes are different from other E/M services.

**9.4** Identify factors of E/M codes for emergency services.

**9.5** Explain how critical care services are reported.

**9.6** Describe factors that determine subcategories of E/M services in special settings.

**9.7** Explain how time is calculated and used to report prolonged services.

**9.8** Identify the factors that determine which E/M codes are reported for case management and care plan oversight services.

**9.9** Describe preventive medicine services.

**9.10** Identify elements of telephone, online, and special E/M services.

**9.11** Contrast E/M coding standards for various newborn services.

## Introduction

Selecting the appropriate code to describe evaluation and management (E/M) services provided to patients is often more difficult than selecting codes describing surgical procedures. Procedure code selection involves matching the services provided to the code description to determine which code most accurately describes the actual services. E/M code selection is more complex, involving several key components—history, physical exam, and medical decision making—each of which have four separate levels of service.

In addition, E/M code selection depends on where the services were provided, such as office setting, inpatient hospital setting, emergency department, nursing facility, etc. Each location has different levels of E/M codes, each of which have varying requirements regarding the levels of the key components that must be met to select that code. Some code series require that all three key components meet or exceed the levels in the code description, while other code series only

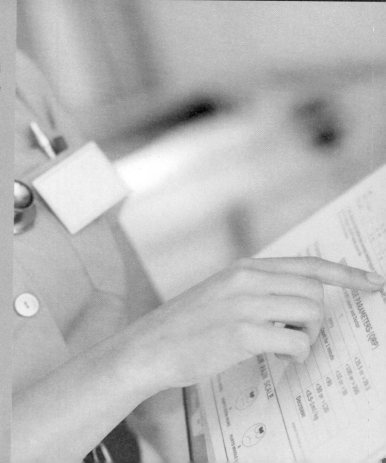

require that two out of three key components meet or exceed the levels in the code description. Contributory factors, such as new versus established patient or initial versus subsequent day, often determine how many key components must be met when selecting the proper code. For some codes the patient's age determines correct code selection. Coders must understand how key components and contributory factors determine the correct E/M code.

## Key Terms

Define each of the following key terms in the space provided.

1. [LO 9.2] Admit/discharge codes _____

_____

2. [LO 9.2] Hospital inpatient services _____

_____

3. [LO 9.2] Hospital observation services _____

_____

4. [LO 9.11] Newborn services _____

_____

5. [LO 9.9] Preventive medicine services _____

_____

6. [LO 9.7] Prolonged services _____

_____

## Exam Review

Select the letter that best completes the statement or answers the question.

1. [LO 9.5] When reporting critical care services, which is more important?
   a. Place of service, such as ER, ICU, or CCU
   b. Level of care first, then place of service
   c. Critical care services are defined by level of care, not place of service
   d. None of these

2. [LO 9.7] Which code(s) report(s) prolonged physician services with direct patient contact for 1 hour and 15 minutes beyond the usual time in the outpatient setting?
   a. 99354
   b. 99355
   c. 99356, 99355
   d. 99354, 99355

3. [LO 9.11] E/M services for the newborn include which of the following?
   a. History and physical on the infant itself
   b. Maternal and infant history and infant physical
   c. Maternal history and physical
   d. Paternal physical

4. [LO 9.8] Which level of codes would you use to report warfarin therapy?
   a. Hypertensive therapy
   b. Laboratory therapy
   c. Anticoagulant therapy
   d. All of these

5. [LO 9.11] What is the duration of time during which a patient is considered a newborn?
   a. First 30 days
   b. First 28 days
   c. First 60 days
   d. First 90 days

6. [LO 9.10] What instructions are provided to a coder in the parenthetical guidance following CPT codes describing telephone services?
   a. Code each 15 minutes of the telephone call.
   b. Do not report certain codes with CPT codes describing telephone calls.
   c. Must also report other appropriate HCPCS codes with telephone calls.
   d. All of these.

7. [LO 9.1] What factor determines whether a patient is considered a new patient?
   a. Patient has never been seen in the office.
   b. Patient has not been seen in past year by any member of the physician group.
   c. Patient has not been seen in three years by any member of the physician group of the same specialty.
   d. Patient has never seen a physician.

8. [LO 9.2] When would it be appropriate to report hospital observation services?
   a. When there is no hospital bed available
   b. When it is not clear that patient should be admitted
   c. Either (a) or (b)
   d. Neither (a) or (b)

9. [LO 9.7] Which of the following services is not described by critical care codes?
   a. Vascular access procedures
   b. Ventilator management
   c. Placement of permanent cardiac pacemaker
   d. Chest x-rays

10. [LO 9.7] What is the most important rule regarding prolonged service codes?
    a. Must report in increments of 1 hour
    b. Must report initial hour then in 15-minute increments
    c. Can never be reported without valid primary E/M code
    d. None of these

11. [LO 9.1] What is the correct code for the office or other outpatient visit of an established patient that may not require the presence of a physician?
    a. 99210
    b. 99211
    c. 99212
    d. 99213

12. [LO 9.2] What is the E/M code used to report the subsequent hospital care of a patient who requires a detailed examination and medical decision making of high complexity?
    a. 99230
    b. 99231
    c. 99232
    d. 99233

13. [LO 9.1] Which code is used to report an office consultation for a patient who requires a comprehensive history, a comprehensive examination, and medical decision making of high complexity?
    a. 99250
    b. 99240
    c. 99245
    d. 99255

14. [LO 9.4] Which E/M code is used to report an emergency department visit with an expanded problem-focused history, an expanded problem-focused examination, and medical decision making of moderate complexity?

   **a.** 99283
   **b.** 99288
   **c.** 99280
   **d.** 99292

15. [LO 9.6] The E/M code used to report the initial nursing facility care of a patient with a detailed history, a comprehensive examination, and medical decision making of low complexity is _____.

   **a.** 99300
   **b.** 99302
   **c.** 99304
   **d.** 99306

16. [LO 9.6] Choose the code used to report nursing facility discharge day management lasting for 45 minutes.

   **a.** 99316
   **b.** 99315
   **c.** 99314
   **d.** 99313

17. [LO 9.6] Which code is used to report the home visit for a new patient with a problem-focused history, a problem-focused examination, and straightforward medical decision making?

   **a.** 99340
   **b.** 99341
   **c.** 99342
   **d.** 99343

18. [LO 9.7] Prolonged evaluation and management services lasting 50 minutes total time before and after direct patient care are reported by code _____.

   **a.** 99354
   **b.** 99358
   **c.** 99355
   **d.** 99357

19. [LO 9.2] The initial hospital care of a patient with a comprehensive history, a comprehensive examination, and straightforward medical decision making is reported with which of the following codes?

   **a.** 99220
   **b.** 99222
   **c.** 99221
   **d.** 99223

20. [LO 9.9] What is the E/M code used to report preventive medicine counseling and risk factor reduction intervention lasting for 15 minutes?

   **a.** 99410
   **b.** 99407
   **c.** 99404
   **d.** 99401

21. [LO 9.8] A 40-minute medical team conference with an interdisciplinary team of healthcare professionals, face to face with the patient and her family, would be reported by code _____.

   **a.** 99366
   **b.** 99364
   **c.** 99362
   **d.** 99360

22. [LO 9.10] Which code describes a work-related examination by an individual other than the treating physician that includes the completion of a medical history commensurate with the patient's condition; the performance of an examination commensurate with the patient's condition; the formulation of a diagnosis, assessment of capabilities and stability, and a calculation of impairment; the development of future medical treatment plan; and the completion of necessary documentation?

   **a.** 99450

   **b.** 99452

   **c.** 99454

   **d.** 99456

23. [LO 9.6] Which code is used to report the home visit of an established patient that requires a detailed interval history and medical decision making of moderate complexity?

   **a.** 99343

   **b.** 99346

   **c.** 99349

   **d.** 99340

24. [LO 9.4] Which E/M code refers to physician direction of emergency medical systems (EMS) emergency care?

   **a.** 99290

   **b.** 99288

   **c.** 99298

   **d.** 99280

25. [LO 9.2] The observation or inpatient hospital care of a patient, including admission and discharge on the same date, which requires a comprehensive history, a comprehensive examination, and medical decision making of high complexity, is reported using code _____.

   **a.** 99230

   **b.** 99320

   **c.** 99236

   **d.** 99362

## Applying Your Skills

Using your CPT manual, assign the appropriate E/M code(s) to report each encounter.

1. [LO 9.3] A patient is admitted to the hospital for complications arising from colon cancer. An oncologist is brought in for a consultation and performs a comprehensive history and examination. His medical decision making is of high complexity. Which code should be used to report this service?

   _____

2. [LO 9.6] An established patient at a rest home develops a significant new problem and requires immediate physician evaluation. His regular physician performs a comprehensive interval history and comprehensive examination. Which code reports this service?

   _____

3. [LO 9.9] If a physician hosts a weekly, hour-long preventive medicine counseling seminar for a group of 10 individuals, which code should be used to reference his services?

   _____

4. [LO 9.11] Larissa exhibits neonatal apnea and respiratory distress in the delivery room. The attending physician provides positive pressure ventilation. Which code should be used to report this procedure?

   _____

5. [LO 9.7] Dr. Donati is asked to monitor the EEG of a patient recovering from brain surgery. Which E/M code is used to report her services?

   _____

   

**6.** [LO 9.11]  Which code is used to report initial inpatient pediatric critical care for a 4-year-old child?

_____

**7.** [LO 9.9]  Forty-two-year-old Claire visits her usual physician for her annual well-woman exam. Which code should her physician use to reference this preventive service?

_____

**8.** [LO 9.10]  Which code is used to report a disability examination that includes measurement of height, weight, and blood pressure; completion of a medical history; collection of blood for testing; and completion of necessary documentation?

_____

**9.** [LO 9.6]  Dr. Stevenson makes a house visit to her regular patient, Mr. Morgan. She performs a comprehensive examination and, due to Mr. Morgan's unstable health, is required to make medical decisions of high complexity. Which code is used to report this visit?

_____

**10.** [LO 9.9]  Which code is used to reference initial comprehensive preventive medicine visit for a 15-year-old adolescent?

_____

**11.** [LO 9.2]  Thomas has been in the hospital for two days and has not shown adequate response to his treatment. His physician performs an expanded problem-focused examination and is required to make medical decisions of moderate complexity. Which code should be used to report his physician's services?

_____

**12.** [LO 9.11]  Alex is born prematurely and requires critical care for three days following his birth. Which code(s) should be used, per day, to report these services?

_____

**13.** [LO 9.6]  Dr. Jaycees visits a new patient at a boarding house who presents with flu-like symptoms. He performs a problem-focused history and examination, and straightforward medical decision making is required. Which code is used to report his services?

_____

**14.** [LO 9.4]  Alice is brought to the emergency room after a car accident. The ER attending physician performs a detailed history and examination. Her medical decision making is of moderate complexity as Alice's wounds, while severe, are not life-threatening. Which code is appropriate to report these services?

_____

**15.** [LO 9.8]  Which code should be used to report the services of a physician supervising the care plan of a hospice patient, involving development of care plans, communication, and adjustment of medical therapy, if the physician spends approximately 25 minutes performing these services?

_____

## Case Studies

For each of the following scenarios, assign the appropriate E/M code(s).

**1.** [LO 9.8]  Edith is admitted to Sunrise Nursing Home with a diagnosis of advanced senile dementia, Alzheimer's, malignant hypertension, and anemia. The admitting physician spends 45 minutes at her bedside and performs a comprehensive history and examination with high-complexity decision making. Code the E/M visit.

_____

**2.** [LO 9.4]  Mr. Green was stung by a hornet and experienced a severe allergic reaction. He was seen in the emergency room by Dr. Kato, who performed a detailed history and physical examination and made medical decisions of moderate complexity. What is the E/M code?

_____

**3.** [LO 9.1] While fishing with his grandfather, Antonio was hooked through the ear by a used fish hook. After removing the hook, Antonio went to his family physician for a tetanus injection, which was administered by the office nurse without Antonio seeing the physician. Which E/M code describes this service?

_____

**4.** [LO 9.4] Joshua was hunting in the woods and tripped and fell into the river. He presented to the emergency room with acute hypothermia and frostbite of his fingers. The physician admitting him for observation performed a comprehensive history and physical examination. Medical decision making was of low complexity. Which E/M code describes these services?

_____

**5.** [LO 9.1] While playing baseball, Zach was injured by a wild pitch that fractured his zygomatic process. He presented to the physician's office as a new patient. The physician performed an expanded problem-focused history and exam with straightforward medical decision making. What is the E/M code?

_____

**6.** [LO 9.9] Melissa presents to her family physician for a second round of hepatitis B immunization injections. She is 23 years old. What is the E/M code?

_____

**7.** [LO 9.2] Jesse was discharged from the hospital after an overnight stay for a head injury. The discharge took less than 30 minutes. Which E/M code describes the discharge services?

_____

**8.** [LO 9.1] Ella experiences headache and earache due to otitis media. She is examined by her family physician and is treated with antibiotics. What is the E/M code for the office visit?

_____

**9.** [LO 9.1] Eric went to his doctor's office for examination and repair of severe lacerations to his face and neck after his PlayStation blew up in his face. This required a detailed history and examination with medical decision making of moderate complexity. What is the E/M code?

_____

**10.** [LO 9.6] Dr. Jones performs a house call for Gladys Townsend, a new patient, to examine her for possible pneumonia. He performs a detailed history and physical exam with medical decision making of moderate complexity. What is the E/M code?

_____

## Thinking It Through

Using your critical thinking skills, answer the following questions.

**1.** [LO 9.1, 9.2, 9.5] Why is it important for the coder to know the location where E/M services were provided to a patient? Is this always true? Why or why not?

_____

_____

_____

**2.** [LO 9.4] What is the difference between new and established patients in the context of emergency department E/M services?

_____

_____

_____

**3.** [LO 9.2] A patient can be considered a "new" patient even with his or her longtime family physician. How is this possible? Why is this important when coding?

_____

_____

_____

_____

**4.** [LO 9.3] Consultation services are reported in a variety of ways. Describe a situation in which a consultation is provided but not reported with consultation codes.

_____

_____

_____

_____

**5.** [LO 9.10] A physician using the Internet to respond to a patient would report that service with which code? What limit is placed on how often a physician can report that code? Are there exceptions to any limit that exists? Explain the main reason for your answer.

_____

_____

_____

_____

## Learning Outcomes

*After completing this chapter, students should be able to:*

**10.1** Select anesthesia codes based on surgical procedures.

**10.2** Report anesthesia time.

**10.3** Use anesthesia modifiers and add-on codes.

**10.4** Calculate the total number of anesthesia units for services provided.

**10.5** Select anesthesia codes for surgical procedures on specific body parts.

**10.6** Choose anesthesia codes for specific procedures.

## Introduction

Reporting anesthesia services is different from reporting other services provided to patients. The correct anesthesia code does not depend on the services the anesthesia provider performs on the patient, but on the procedures being performed by other providers, such as surgeons, that make the anesthesia necessary.

Most anesthesia codes are organized based on anatomical structures involved in the surgical procedure performed. Some anesthesia codes are organized by the type of procedure, rather than on the anatomical location on which the procedure is performed, such as anesthesia for radiological procedures or the treatment of burns. Each anesthesia code has a value that is referred to as the number of base units.

Anesthesia services also differ from other procedures in that the time the anesthesia services are provided is reported separately from the code that describes the anesthesia. Time units are assigned to each anesthetic based on the total time the services are provided. In addition to the base units and anesthesia time, anesthesia units may be added based on the general overall health of the patient and special qualifying circumstances, such as extreme age or the intentional use of hypothermia or hypotension during the anesthesia.

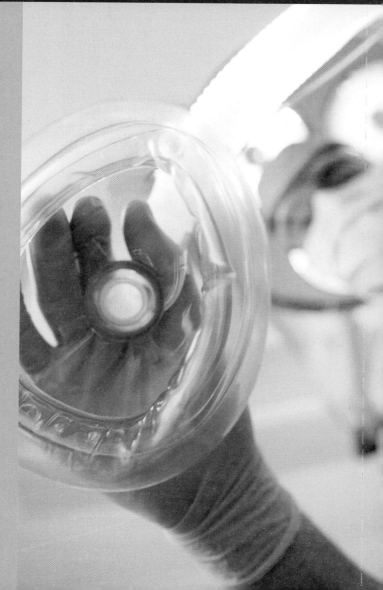

# Key Terms

Define each of the following key terms in the space provided.

**1.** [LO 10.3] Anesthesiologist _____

_____

**2.** [LO 10.3] Certified registered nurse anesthetist _____

_____

**3.** [LO 10.3] Anesthesia assistant _____

_____

**4.** [LO 10.1] General anesthesia _____

_____

**5.** [LO 10.1] Regional anesthesia _____

_____

**6.** [LO 10.1] Local anesthesia _____

_____

**7.** [LO 10.3] Monitored anesthesia care _____

_____

**8.** [LO 10.1] American Society of Anesthesiologists _____

_____

**9.** [LO 10.1] Analgesia _____

_____

**10.** [LO 10.3] Qualifying circumstances add-on code _____

_____

# Exam Review

Select the letter that best completes the statement or answers the question.

**1.** [LO 10.1] Which of the following are included in the CPT code descriptions of anesthesia services?
   **a.** The procedures performed that make anesthesia necessary
   **b.** The general health status of the patient
   **c.** Whether the anesthesia is general, regional, local, and/or monitored anesthesia care
   **d.** Both (*a*) and (*b*)

**2.** [LO 10.1] Which of the following statements is true regarding anesthesia services?
   **a.** Anesthesia services must be provided by an anesthesiologist.
   **b.** Payment is contingent upon the type of anesthesia administered.
   **c.** Payment is not contingent upon the type of anesthesia administered.
   **d.** More than one anesthesia code must be used to describe anesthesia services.

**3.** [LO 10.1] Surgical procedures described by a single anesthesia CPT code are often similar to one another with respect to which of the following criteria?
   **a.** Anticipated blood loss
   **b.** Typical need for fluid or blood replacement
   **c.** Affects on blood pressure and other physiological parameters
   **d.** All of these

4. [LO 10.1] Which of the following can be said about the anesthesia codes with the *not otherwise specified* notation?
   a. Other anesthesia codes may describe the services better.
   b. Typical anesthesia services for surgery on a particular body part are described in general anatomical terms with a *not otherwise specified* notation.
   c. A single anesthesia code may be used to describe anesthesia for a number of different surgical procedures that involve a general area of the body or specific body part.
   d. All of these.

5. [LO 10.1] Which of the following statements is true regarding anesthesia codes?
   a. Few codes need to be used because the codes share common factors that relate to a number of surgical procedures.
   b. There is a bias in choosing one anesthesia code over another.
   c. Fees for anesthesia services depend on the type of anesthetic.
   d. The underlying procedure is independent of the anesthesia administered for it.

6. [LO 10.2] Which of the following statements is *not* true regarding anesthesia time units?
   a. Time units are often calculated on the basis of 15-minute intervals.
   b. Some portion of the next time unit is counted as a whole unit, but that portion varies among payers.
   c. Anesthesia time may be reported in minutes.
   d. Anesthesia time is the same among all payers.

7. [LO 10.2] What is the proper procedure for an insurance carrier to follow when calculating payment for anesthesia services?
   a. Conversion of anesthesia time into units for payment purposes
   b. Calculation of time units based upon 15 minutes
   c. Assignment of a P-status modifier
   d. Denial of the claim until documentation is sent

8. [LO 10.2] What are the primary coding activities necessary for reporting anesthesia services?
   a. Selecting the appropriate anesthesia CPT code
   b. Calculating anesthesia time
   c. Assigning anesthesia modifiers
   d. All of these

9. [LO 10.3] Which of the following is the purpose of physical status modifiers?
   a. To describe the general overall health of the patient
   b. To describe the credentials of the individual providing the anesthetic
   c. To describe reasons for the monitored anesthesia care (MAC)
   d. All of these

10. [LO 10.3] Which of the following actions should a medical coder take when coding for anesthesia?
    a. Always append a P-status modifier.
    b. Add qualifying circumstances to every anesthesia claim.
    c. Identify the professional credentials of anesthesia providers who are physicians.
    d. Only append a P-status modifier if you know it is reimbursable.

11. [LO 10.3] Which codes should be used to identify the professional credentials of anesthesia providers?
    a. HCPCS modifiers
    b. CPT modifiers
    c. P-status modifiers
    d. Qualifying circumstances

12. [LO 10.2, 10.3] Which of the following is true about P-status modifiers?
    a. Patients with physical status P1 or P2 do not pose significant additional anesthesia risks to justify additional payments.
    b. P6 is used to identify a brain-dead patient undergoing organ donation procedures.
    c. CPT code 01990 does not require a P-status modifier.
    d. All of these.

**13.** [LO 10.6] Which of the following radiological procedures typically do not require anesthesia?

  **a.** X-rays to visualize a body part
  **b.** Procedures that cause sufficient discomfort
  **c.** Anesthesia for cardiac catheterization
  **d.** Anesthesia for diagnostic venography

**14.** [LO 10.6] How many codes are available to describe anesthesia for the treatment of burns?

  **a.** Hundreds
  **b.** Two
  **c.** One per body area
  **d.** Two and one add-on code

**15.** [LO 10.6] Which of the following is the correct way to code for a cesarean section after a trial of labor?

  **a.** A base code is used to describe the labor analgesia and an add-on code to report the cesarean section.
  **b.** Code 01961 anesthesia for cesarean section only
  **c.** Codes 01960 and 01961
  **d.** An add-on code is used to report the labor analgesia and the cesarean section.

**16.** [LO 10.3] Which of the following is a HCPCS modifier for monitored anesthesia services?

  **a.** AD
  **b.** QP
  **c.** QS
  **d.** QY

**17.** [LO 10.3] Which of the following is the correct modifier for monitored anesthesia care (MAC) for a patient with a history of severe cardiopulmonary disease?

  **a.** CPT modifier
  **b.** G9
  **c.** QX
  **d.** 23

**18.** [LO 10.3] Which of the following is an example of anesthesia modifiers that identify the professional credentials of professionals who provide anesthesia services?

  **a.** AA, GC, and BB
  **b.** AA, AD, GC, and GK
  **c.** QX, QY, and QZ
  **d.** QX, QY, AA, and AC

**19.** [LO 10.3] Which of the following codes for qualifying circumstances is appropriate to describe a patient with induced decreased blood pressure levels that can potentially cause complications?

  **a.** 99140
  **b.** 99135
  **c.** 99100
  **d.** 99116

**20.** [LO 10.4] Which of the following is the basic formula for calculating total anesthesia units?

  **a.** B × T × M = total anesthesia units
  **b.** B + T + M + QC = total anesthesia units
  **c.** B + T + M = total anesthesia units
  **d.** B × T × QC × M = total anesthesia units

**21.** [LO 10.4] Which of the following should be reported for all anesthesia services?

  **a.** Qualifying circumstances and modifying factors
  **b.** Base units, qualifying circumstances, and modifying factors
  **c.** Base units, time units, and physical status modifiers
  **d.** Qualifying circumstances, base units, and time units

22. [LO 10.3] Which of the following identifies anesthesia administered by a certified registered nurse anesthetist (CRNA) under the supervision of a physician?
    a. QZ
    b. QS
    c. QY
    d. QX

23. [LO 10.3] Which of the following is the appropriate modifier to describe medical supervision by a physician for more than four concurrent anesthesia services?
    a. AA
    b. 23
    c. AD
    d. QK

24. [LO 10.3] The appropriate CPT modifier for reporting anesthesia that is greater than that usually required for the listed procedure is _____.
    a. 23
    b. AD
    c. 22
    d. QK

25. [LO 10.3] Anesthesia administered by a surgeon is reported with code _____.
    a. 47
    b. AD
    c. QS
    d. 59

26. [LO 10.5] Anesthesia for procedures on which of the following structures is described by CPT codes in the Intrathoracic section of anesthesia codes, 00500–00580?
    a. Heart and lungs
    b. Upper abdomen
    c. Access to the central venous system
    d. Both (a) and (c)

27. [LO 10.5] Which of the following code ranges is used to report anesthesia for diagnostic and therapeutic nerve blocks and injections?
    a. 00600–00670
    b. 01991–01992
    c. 00530–00537
    d. 00902–00952

28. [LO 10.5] Which of the following codes is appropriate for a flexible esophagoscopy for the removal of a foreign body?
    a. 00790
    b. 00800
    c. 00740
    d. 00840

29. [LO 10.3] The appropriate modifier for two, three, or four concurrent anesthesia procedures under the direction of qualified individuals is _____.
    a. QS
    b. AD
    c. QK
    d. AA

**30.** [LO 10.5] The anesthesia code for diagnostic arteriography/venography is _____.

    **a.** 01916

    **b.** 00914

    **c.** 01112

    **d.** 00938

## Applying Your Skills

Using your CPT manual, assign the appropriate code(s) to each service.

**1.** [LO 10.5] Anesthesia for a cranioplasty or elevation of depressed skull fracture, extradural. _____

**2.** [LO 10.5] Jay is anesthetized for procedures on his heart, pericardial sac, and the great vessels of his chest. He does not require a pump oxygenator during surgery. _____

**3.** [LO 10.5] Anesthesia for any patient under 1 year of age for a procedure on the larynx and trachea. _____

**4.** [LO 10.5] Anesthesia for upper gastrointestinal endoscopic procedures, when the endoscope is introduced proximal to duodenum. _____

**5.** [LO 10.5] Anesthesia for a radical prostatectomy (suprapubic, retropubic). _____

**6.** [LO 10.5] Anesthesia for hysteroscopy and/or hysterosalpingography procedures. _____

**7.** [LO 10.5] Anesthesia for closed procedures involving the symphysis pubis and sacroiliac joint. _____

**8.** [LO 10.5] A patient requires a femoral artery embolectomy and will have anesthesia for this procedure. _____

**9.** [LO 10.5] Anesthesia for a popliteal thromboendarterectomy, with or without a patch graft. _____

**10.** [LO 10.5] Susie has fractured her lower leg and is anesthetized while the cast is applied. _____

**11.** [LO 10.5] Anesthesia for an interthoracoscapular (forequarter) amputation. _____

**12.** [LO 10.5] Anesthesia for open or surgical arthroscopic procedures of the elbow, not otherwise specified. _____

**13.** [LO 10.5] Arthur requires anesthesia for diagnostic arthroscopic procedures on his wrist. _____

**14.** [LO 10.6] Anesthesia for a patient undergoing cardiac catheterization, including coronary angiography and ventriculography. _____

**15.** [LO 10.6] Mrs. Sanchez is admitted to the hospital for a planned vaginal delivery. What code should be used to document the epidural labor analgesia/anesthesia she is given during the labor and delivery? _____

## Case Studies

For each of the following scenarios, assign the appropriate anesthesia code(s).

**1.** [LO 10.5] A tennis player has been having pain, swelling, and popping of the knee. Her orthopedic surgeon discovers a torn medial meniscus of the knee and performs an arthroscopic repair of the meniscus. Which CPT code describes the anesthesia for this procedure? _____

**2.** [LO 10.5] A 36-year-old patient with a history of Hashimoto thyroiditis has been having increased difficulty swallowing (dysphagia). She examines her throat area and discovers an unusual nodule on her neck. She sees her primary care physician, who refers her to Dr. Mattias, an endocrinologist. Dr. Mattias orders an ultrasound-guided fine needle aspiration for biopsy. A malignant neoplasm of the thyroid is discovered, for which excision is necessary. Report the anesthesia for the thyroidectomy. _____

**3.** [LO 10.6] Mallory has been receiving routine obstetrical care and has been in labor for 27 hours. She has only dilated 2 cm, and labor is further induced with Pitocin to increase dilation and uterine contractions. Mallory's water is broken, and forceps delivery is attempted when it is discovered that the baby is breech. This results in an immediate cesarean section. Identify the code(s) describing the anesthesia services. _____

4. [LO 10.5] Painter Vincent van Gogh's signs of mental illness may have been due to cadmium exposure from the bright pigments in the orange and red paints he used. Likewise, a lifelong artist who works with cadmium paints could also be at risk for kidney cancer. In the event of renal neoplasm requiring a laparoscopic removal of the kidney, report the anesthesia for this service. _____

5. [LO 10.6] Michael, now 6, was born with tetralogy of Fallot. After numerous surgeries to correct this condition, pulmonary stenosis occurs. As a result, blood flow from the right ventricle of the heart is obstructed, causing a reduction in blood flow to the lungs. Pulmonary artery dilation is necessary and is performed by the insertion of a balloon catheter through the skin. Report the anesthesia service. _____

6. [LO 10.5] A 62-year-old male developed cardiac arrhythmia and displays bradycardia on an EKG. He requires a permanent transvenous pacemaker insertion. The subclavian vein was accessed, and a pulse generator pocket was formed to accommodate the pacemaker. Report the anesthesia administered to perform this procedure. _____

7. [LO 10.5] Samuel is diagnosed with prostate cancer and undergoes a retropubic radical prostatectomy. The surgeon also performs lymph node biopsies. Identify the CPT codes describing the anesthesia. _____

8. [LO 10.5] Joey, a professional ice hockey player, was struck by a defenseman from the opposing team, fracturing his clavicle. He was taken to the emergency room. Assign the appropriate CPT codes for the anesthesia administered for the repair of the fracture. _____

9. [LO 10.5] A medical school graduate spends the summer in the rural countryside of Austria. Upon her return to the United States to complete her medical residency, she begins experiencing abdominal pain and diarrhea. She sees her gastroenterologist who discovers eosinophilia in response to an antigen/allergen. A CT scan of the liver reveals that she has echinococcal parasitic cysts of the liver. The condition has progressed to the point that a partial hepatectomy is required. Assign the appropriate CPT codes for the anesthesia required to perform the procedure. _____

10. [LO 10.5] A patient has had a pancreatic pseudocyst for several years with chronic pain. Symptoms have worsened and are unresponsive to conservative therapy. The surgeon recommends a total pancreatectomy with autologous pancreatic islet cell transplant to avoid the complication of surgically induced diabetes. Report the anesthesia required to perform this procedure. _____

## Thinking It Through

Using your critical-thinking skills, answer the questions below.

1. [LO 10.1] Identify the professionals who deliver anesthesia. Provide a brief description of each one's role.

_____

_____

_____

_____

2. [LO 10.1] Other than the administration of anesthesia, identify services provided by anesthesia providers?

_____

_____

_____

_____

3. [LO 10.1] Identify and describe the four major types of anesthesia that may be administered.

_____

_____

_____

_____

**4.** [LO 10.2, 10.3, 10.4]  What steps should a coder take to determine the correct CPT code describing an anesthesia procedure?

_____

_____

_____

_____

**5.** [LO 10.4]  How does a coder calculate the number of anesthesia units?

_____

_____

_____

_____

# 11 RADIOLOGY SERVICES

## Learning Outcomes

*After completing this chapter, students should be able to:*

**11.1** Define positions, projections, and planes in terms of radiology services.

**11.2** Explain the process for reporting radiology services.

**11.3** Use modifiers with radiology CPT codes.

**11.4** Discuss parameters surrounding CPT coding for various radiology services.

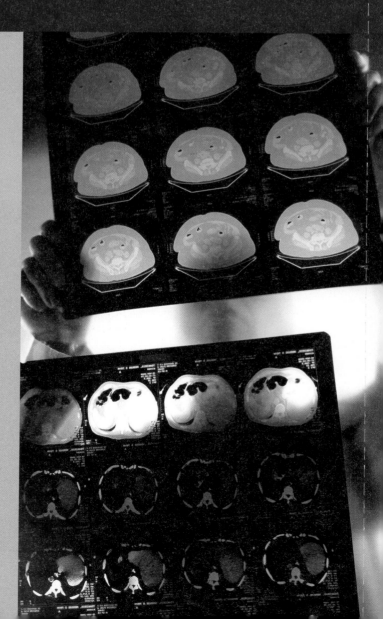

## Introduction

Radiology encompasses a broad array of services, ranging from a simple x-ray using techniques that are over a century old to the most modern scans using computers combined with radiation beams, magnetic fields, and radioactive substances. Modern scans produce images of what is happening deep inside the patient's body down to the level of cellular activity. CPT codes describing these services are included in the 70000 series.

The diagnostic radiology or diagnostic imaging section of the 70000 series includes codes describing x-rays, CT scans, MRIs, and MRAs. This section is subdivided by anatomical location. Separate sections include codes describing ultrasound procedures, radiological guidance, mammography, and bone and joint studies. Radiation oncology and nuclear medicine studies are described in separate sections.

Most radiological procedures include professional and technical components, reported with modifiers 26 and TC, respectively. Some radiology codes include the term "radiological supervision and interpretation" in their code descriptors. These codes describe professional radiological services performed as part of other services and do not require modifier 26.

# Key Terms

Define each of the following key terms in the space provided.

**1.** [LO 11.1]  Anteroposterior (AP) _____

_____

**2.** [LO 11.1]  Computed tomography (CT) _____

_____

**3.** [LO 11.2]  Contrast material _____

_____

**4.** [LO 11.1]  Coronal plane _____

_____

**5.** [LO 11.1]  Decubitus _____

_____

**6.** [LO 11.1]  Digital x-ray system _____

_____

**7.** [LO 11.1]  Fluoroscopy _____

_____

**8.** [LO 11.1]  Left lateral decubitus _____

_____

**9.** [LO 11.1]  Magnetic resonance imaging (MRI) _____

_____

**10.** [LO 11.4]  Mammography _____

_____

**11.** [LO 11.3]  Modifier 26 _____

_____

**12.** [LO 11.3]  Modifier TC _____

_____

**13.** [LO 11.1]  Nuclear medicine _____

_____

**14.** [LO 11.1]  Oblique _____

_____

**15.** [LO 11.1]  Posteroanterior (PA) _____

_____

**16.** [LO 11.1]  Prone _____

_____

**17.** [LO 11.2]  Radiological supervision and interpretation _____

_____

**18.** [LO 11.1]  Right lateral decubitus _____

_____

**19.** [LO 11.1]  Sagittal plane _____

_____

**20.** [LO 11.1] Standing _____

_____

**21.** [LO 11.1] Supine _____

_____

**22.** [LO 11.1] Tomogram _____

_____

**23.** [LO 11.1] Transverse plane _____

_____

**24.** [LO 11.1] Ultrasound _____

_____

**25.** [LO 11.1] X-ray film _____

_____

# Exam Review

Select the letter that best describes the statement or answers the question.

**1.** [LO 11.1] The radiographic projection terminology is defined by _____.
   **a.** Where the radiation beam exits and enters the body
   **b.** The part of the body against the film plate
   **c.** Where the radiation beam enters and exits the body
   **d.** The direction the radiation beam is pointed in the x-ray room

**2.** [LO 11.1] Which imaging modality combines images into a composite view using computers?
   **a.** MRI
   **b.** CT
   **c.** MRI and CT
   **d.** Neither MRI nor CT

**3.** [LO 11.1] Which is not an anatomical position during diagnostic radiographic imaging?
   **a.** Supine
   **b.** Transverse
   **c.** Lateral decubitus
   **d.** Prone

**4.** [LO 11.2] Which of the following is an example of a situation where "radiological supervision and interpretation" or "component coding" would be used?
   **a.** A radiologist places a catheter for contrast injection and also reads the x-rays.
   **b.** A radiologist takes a chest x-ray and reads it.
   **c.** A radiologist reads prereduction and postreduction arm fracture x-rays.
   **d.** A radiologist gives sedation and performs an x-ray.

**5.** [LO 11.2] A coder should use an "unlisted" radiology CPT code when _____.
   **a.** The type of radiology modality performed is not specified
   **b.** Extra time, effort, and equipment are necessary for a radiology service
   **c.** A radiologist performs both the supervision and interpretation of a radiology service
   **d.** A particular radiology service provided is not described by a specific CPT code

**6.** [LO 11.2]  Each of the following might require use of a 59 modifier except _____.

   **a.** Separate procedure done on a different body part
   **b.** Separate procedure done on a different day
   **c.** Separate procedure done during a different surgical session, same day
   **d.** Separate procedure performed during a different surgical procedure, same day

**7.** [LO 11.3]  A radiologist owns a freestanding imaging facility which takes a chest x-ray of a patient that is read by the radiologist. Which modifiers would best be used for the coding of this chest x-ray service?

   **a.** 26 and TC
   **b.** 26 or TC
   **c.** No modifiers
   **d.** TC only

**8.** [LO 11.3]  Which combination of radiology services would require use of a 50 modifier?

   **a.** AP x-ray view of left hand and lateral view x-ray of right hand
   **b.** AP and lateral view x-ray of left hand, repeated
   **c.** AP and lateral view x-ray of left hand, before and after fracture reduction
   **d.** AP and lateral view x-ray of left hand and AP and lateral view x-ray of right hand

**9.** [LO 11.4]  Which of the following is not a main division of the radiology CPT codes?

   **a.** Radiologic guidance
   **b.** Endoscopic imaging
   **c.** Breast mammography
   **d.** Nuclear medicine

**10.** [LO 11.4]  The Diagnostic Radiology section is categorized primarily by _____.

   **a.** Degree of invasiveness of the study
   **b.** Use of contrast
   **c.** Anatomical region
   **d.** Intensity of radiation used for study

**11.** [LO 11.4]  Which of the following modalities is never used for radiological guidance for procedures?

   **a.** Radiation oncology
   **b.** Ultrasound
   **c.** CT
   **d.** Fluoroscopy

**12.** [LO 11.4]  A valid "complete" diagnostic ultrasound of a given anatomical area specified in a CPT code must include documentation of _____.

   **a.** Each element of the exam viewed in at least two projections
   **b.** Biometric data and the permanent ultrasound images
   **c.** Each required element listed by the anatomical subsection
   **d.** Indication of whether pathology was found or not

**13.** [LO 11.4]  A bone density test is an example of _____.

   **a.** Diagnostic radiology
   **b.** Nuclear medicine
   **c.** Diagnostic ultrasound
   **d.** Bone/joint study

**14.** [LO 11.4]  Which of the following is not an example of a radiation oncology service?

   **a.** Oral administration of radioactive medications to treat thyroid cancer
   **b.** Initial brachytherapy with radioactive seeds to treat prostate cancer
   **c.** Follow-up PET scan to determine decrease in tumor size after treatment
   **d.** Therapeutic radiology treatment planning

15. [LO 11.4] Which is not a valid route of administration for a radiopharmaceutical agent?
    a. Intra-articular
    b. Interstitial
    c. External beam
    d. Intravenous

16. [LO 11.4] A patient with headache undergoes a CT scan of the brain without contrast. While the patient is still in the CT scanner, the radiologist notes an irregular area in the cerebellum and performs more CT images of the brain with contrast to better delineate the area. Report code(s) _____.
    a. 70450
    b. 70460
    c. 70450 and 70460
    d. 70470

17. [LO 11.4] A patient has a two-view x-ray of the paranasal sinuses documented by the radiologist as "complete sinus study—all findings normal." Report code(s) _____.
    a. 70220
    b. 70210
    c. 70220-52
    d. 70220 and 70210

18. [LO 11.4] A pediatrician is concerned about his patient's bowlegged appearance and orders an x-ray of a 5-year-old girl's knees while standing. Seeking to minimize radiation and to assess symmetry, the pediatrician orders only one view from the front. Reports should have code _____.
    a. 73560
    b. 73560-50
    c. 73565
    d. 77072

19. [LO 11.4] Mrs. Ballard's physician is worried that she may be prone to spine and hip fractures and has her undergo a DXA scan of her spine to check for osteoporosis. What is the code?
    a. 77080
    b. 77082
    c. 77074
    d. 77081

20. [LO 11.4] A patient with chest pain is admitted through the emergency department and undergoes a SPECT scan stress test with quantitative wall motion study to assess myocardial damage. Report this test with code(s) _____.
    a. 78451
    b. 78452
    c. 78466
    d. 78468

21. [LO 11.4] Mrs. Sanchez comes into her obstetrician's office the first time for a high-risk twin pregnancy and has a detailed transabdominal ultrasound of herself and the anatomy of both fetuses, real time with image documentation. Which code(s) should be used to report the procedure?
    a. 76811 and 76814
    b. 76815
    c. 76815 and 76815-59
    d. 76811 and 76812

22. [LO 11.4] Melanie, an infant with clicking hips, undergoes an ultrasound of her hips to check for dislocation while her pediatrician manipulates the joints to replicate the clicking. What is the code?

   **a.** 77077
   **b.** 76885
   **c.** 76886
   **d.** 73520

23. [LO 11.4] A patient with a single breast mass is scheduled for a lumpectomy. Before going to the operating room, she is first seen in radiology for mammographic needle localization and wire placement so the surgeon can locate the mass during surgery. For the radiological guidance only, select the code _____.

   **a.** 77032
   **b.** 77031
   **c.** 77055
   **d.** 77051

24. [LO 11.4] A patient who has just had a cancerous thyroid gland removed has a nuclear medicine imaging scan to assess her whole body for metastases. Report code _____.

   **a.** 78020
   **b.** 78800
   **c.** 78018
   **d.** 77074

25. [LO 11.4] A patient comes to the emergency department with a pulsatile mass in his abdomen. To check for aortic aneurysm, the physician orders a CT angiogram of the abdomen only, with contrast given intravenously. Report code _____.

   **a.** 74185
   **b.** 74175
   **c.** 75635
   **d.** 75630

26. [LO 11.4] Adrian presents with a blast injury to his hand and undergoes a diagnostic angiography of his left hand to visualize the arterial supply prior to reconstruction of his thumb. No intervention is performed at the time of the study. What is the code?

   **a.** 75716
   **b.** 75820
   **c.** 75801
   **d.** 75710

27. [LO 11.4] A metalworker is sent for an ultrasound of his right eye to be assessed for a foreign body. What is the code?

   **a.** 76519
   **b.** 76529
   **c.** 70030
   **d.** 70480

28. [LO 11.4] A child with abdominal pain undergoes a contrast enema to reduce an intussusception of her intestine. What is the code?

   **a.** 74250
   **b.** 74270
   **c.** 74283
   **d.** No radiology code assigned in this case

29. [LO 11.4] A patient with suspected stroke has an MRA (magnetic resonance angiography) of his head and neck, with and without contrast. Report code(s) _____.

   **a.** 70546 and 70549
   **b.** 70545 and 70548
   **c.** 70496 and 70498
   **d.** 70543

30. [LO 11.4] A patient is having low back pain after a car accident and has a two-view x-ray of his lower back. Report code _____.

   a. 72110
   b. 72070
   c. 72131
   d. 72100

## Applying Your Skills

Using your CPT manual, provide codes for the following radiological procedures. Include any necessary modifiers. In some cases, more than one code is required.

1. [LO 11.4] MRI of the cervical spine without contrast. _____

2. [LO 11.4] X-rays of femur, two views. _____

3. [LO 11.4] CT of abdomen, with and without contrast. _____

4. [LO 11.4] CT guidance for placement of radiation therapy fields. _____

5. [LO 11.4] Radiation beam therapy, single treatment area, 15 MeV. _____

6. [LO 11.4] Thyroid uptake study, with stimulation. _____

7. [LO 11.4] Liver SPECT scan with vascular flow study. _____

8. [LO 11.4] Voiding cystogram ureteral reflux study with a bladder residual study. _____

9. [LO 11.4] Radiopharmaceutical therapy, intracavitary administration, after a breast lumpectomy. _____

10. [LO 11.4] A pregnant woman has a first-trimester ultrasound of twin intrauterine gestations to measure fetal nuchal translucency to screen for Down syndrome. _____

11. [LO 11.4] Intravenous pyelogram. _____

12. [LO 11.4] Angiography of superior mesenteric and inferior mesenteric arteries (supervision and interpretation only). _____

13. [LO 11.4] Andrew injures his shoulder, and a four-view x-ray is ordered to determine the extent of the damage. _____

14. [LO 11.4] Posterior fossa myelogram. _____

15. [LO 11.4] Ultrasound guidance for pericardiocentesis. _____

## Case Studies

For each of the following scenarios, assign the appropriate CPT code(s).

1. [LO 11.4] Elizabeth is seen in the emergency department for the gradual onset of a painless swelling under her jaw. The attending physician thinks she might have a salivary gland blocked by a stone and orders an x-ray. After a negative study, the physician then orders a CT scan of the neck soft tissues with contrast to assess for tumors or other causes. Code the radiology procedures.

   _____

2. [LO 11.4] A patient is seen by a maxillofacial specialist for nighttime oral pain and a feeling of locking in his jaw area. To check for asymmetry and other disorders of the teeth, mandible, and temporomandibular joints, the physician orders an orthopantogram and dedicated views of both TMJs. Which code(s) should be used to report the procedures?

   _____

**3.** [LO 11.4]  Rick has been experiencing chronic back pain and is sent for x-rays of his upper and lower back. Two views of the thoracic spine and two views of the lumbosacral spine are obtained. Findings of mild scoliosis and disk degeneration are noted. Report codes for these studies.

_____

**4.** [LO 11.4]  Alison, a patient with abdominal pain, is seen by her family doctor and sent for a noncontrast CT scan of her abdomen. The next day the radiologist reads the study and recalls the patient to have a repeat CT scan of her abdomen with contrast. What are the codes for all radiological services rendered?

_____

**5.** [LO 11.4]  An infant with congenital abnormalities is being worked up for gradual renal failure. She has an intravenous pyelogram (IVP), which shows a blockage of the left ureter and massive hydronephrosis requiring the interventional radiologist to place a percutaneous drainage catheter into the renal pelvis to decompress the kidney. Report all radiology and radiological supervision and interpretation codes.

_____

**6.** [LO 11.4]  Liam develops shortness of breath after an operation. His surgeon suspects a pulmonary embolus (PE). A ventilation-perfusion (V/Q) scan is ordered first, but the results are indeterminate. A CT angiogram is performed and does show a small PE in the left lung. Report codes for all radiological services.

_____

**7.** [LO 11.4]  A patient with prostate cancer undergoes ultrasound-guided complex placement of 120 iodine-131 interstitial brachytherapy seeds into the prostate gland. Which code(s) should be used to report services?

_____

**8.** [LO 11.4]  A toddler is brought to the pediatrician's office by child protective services with a suspicion of child abuse. A "babygram," or infant osseous survey, is performed to screen for skeletal injury. A healing fracture of the left humerus is noted, and two dedicated views of the left arm are taken to determine the extent. Report codes for all procedures.

_____

**9.** [LO 11.4]  Nelson presents to the emergency room with blunt force trauma to the chest and is assessed for internal injuries with a chest ultrasound. This study shows a pericardial hemorrhage with tamponade. The patient is taken immediately to the OR for ultrasound-guided pericardiocentesis. Report codes for radiological imaging, supervision, and interpretation.

_____

**10.** [LO 11.4]  Raquel, a patient with breast cancer, is seen in radiology for placement of a Port-a-Cath central venous access device for chemotherapy as well as stereotactic wire localization of the tumor for surgical excision the next day. What are the codes that describe Raquel's case?

_____

# Thinking It Through

Using your critical-thinking skills, answer the questions below.

**1.** [LO 11.1]  Describe the concept of "projection" as it pertains to the direction of the x-ray beam.

_____

_____

_____

_____

**2.** [LO 11.2]  Define the term "radiological supervision and interpretation." Contrast it with the performance of a procedure from a coding perspective.

_____

_____

_____

_____

**3.** [LO 11.3]  Differentiate between modifiers 26 and TC.

_____

_____

_____

_____

**4.** [LO 11.4]  Describe the difference between a diagnostic imaging study and a radiological guidance procedure.

_____

_____

_____

_____

**5.** [LO 11.4]  What is the difference in the utilization of radiation in the therapeutic categories of radiation oncology and nuclear medicine when compared to the other diagnostic radiology sections?

_____

_____

_____

_____

# GENERAL AND INTEGUMENTARY SYSTEM

## Learning Outcomes

*After completing this module, students should be able to:*

**12.1.1** Identify procedures of the skin and subcutaneous tissues.

**12.1.2** Determine how to group wounds together according to anatomical location and type of closure for reporting purposes.

**12.1.3** Describe the differences between graft, flap, and burn procedures.

**12.1.4** Report tissue destruction of benign and malignant tissues by various techniques.

**12.1.5** Select the appropriate codes for surgical procedures of the breast.

**12.1.6** Code anesthesia services for procedures in the 10000 series.

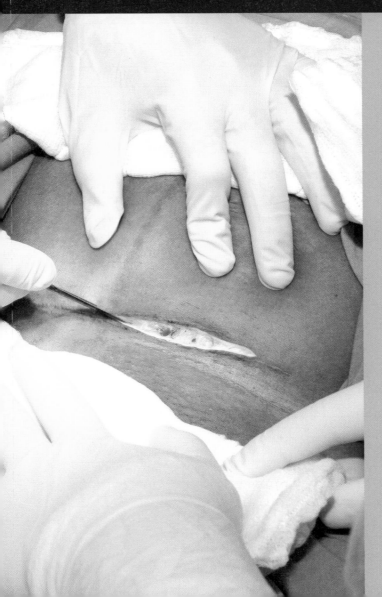

## Introduction

The CPT codes in the 10000 series describe procedures on the integumentary system (skin and subcutaneous tissues), including surgical procedures on the skin; wound repairs; grafts, flaps, and burn procedures; destruction of benign and malignant lesions; and procedures on the breast, including mastectomy and reconstruction.

# Key Terms

Define each of the following key terms in the space provided.

**1.** [LO 12.1.1] Fine needle aspiration _____

_____

**2.** [LO 12.1.1] Incision and drainage (I&D) _____

_____

**3.** [LO 12.1.1] Abscess _____

_____

**4.** [LO 12.1.1] Hematoma _____

_____

**5.** [LO 12.1.1] Debridement _____

_____

**6.** [LO 12.1.1] Necrotizing infection _____

_____

**7.** [LO 12.1.1] Excision _____

_____

**8.** [LO 12.1.1] Hidradenitis _____

_____

**9.** [LO 12.1.2] Simple repair _____

_____

**10.** [LO 12.1.2] Intermediate repair _____

_____

**11.** [LO 12.1.2] Complex repair _____

_____

**12.** [LO 12.1.3] Adjacent tissue transfer _____

_____

**13.** [LO 12.1.3] Autograft _____

_____

**14.** [LO 12.1.3] Allograft _____

_____

**15.** [LO 12.1.3] Xenograft _____

_____

**16.** [LO 12.1.3] Tissue flap _____

_____

**17.** [LO 12.1.4] Mohs micrographic surgery _____

_____

**18.** [LO 12.1.5] Partial mastectomy _____

_____

**19.** [LO 12.1.5] Complete mastectomy _____

_____

**20.** [LO 12.1.5] Radical mastectomy _____

_____

**21.** [LO 12.1.5] Modified radical mastectomy _____

_____

## Exam Review

Select the letter of the answer that best describes the statement or answers the question.

**1.** [LO 12.1.1] The removal of tissue and submitting it for pathological examination is _____.
  **a.** Surgical debridement
  **b.** Excision
  **c.** Biopsy
  **d.** Paring or cutting

**2.** [LO 12.1.1] Skin tags can be removed by _____.
  **a.** Scissoring or any sharp method
  **b.** Chemical or electrosurgical destruction
  **c.** Ligature strangulation
  **d.** All of these

**3.** [LO 12.1.2] Wound repair codes require a coder to know _____.
  **a.** The total length of the repair
  **b.** The anatomical area involved plus the length
  **c.** The total length, the anatomical area, and whether the repair is simple, intermediate, or complex
  **d.** (*a*) and (*b*)

**4.** [LO 12.1.2] According to the CPT manual, complex repair codes _____.
  **a.** Exclude reconstructive procedures or complicated wound closure
  **b.** Include the anatomical site of the repair
  **c.** Include the anatomical site and the length of repair
  **d.** All of these

**5.** [LO 12.1.3] Z-plasty, W-plasty and V-Y plasty are _____.
  **a.** Specialized plastic surgery procedures
  **b.** Performed to transfer or rearrange adjacent tissue
  **c.** Establish a recipient area for a graft
  **d.** None of these

**6.** [LO 12.1.3] Skin grafts _____.
  **a.** Can include human and nonhuman skin
  **b.** Are categorized by anatomical region
  **c.** Can be either autografts, allografts, or xenografts
  **d.** All of these

**7.** [LO 12.1.4] Lesions removed by destruction _____.
  **a.** Should be examined pathologically
  **b.** Are removed via laser, electrosurgery, cryosurgery, and surgical curettement but *not* via chemical treatment
  **c.** Are removed via laser, electrosurgery, cryosurgery, surgical curettement, or by chemical treatment
  **d.** All of these

**8.** [LO 12.1.4] Lesions, if removed by destruction, _____.
  **a.** Are destroyed and counted after surgery
  **b.** Are counted in order to assign the code
  **c.** Are sent for microscopic pathological examination
  **d.** (*b*) and (*c*)

**9.** [LO 12.1.5] Mastectomy codes 19300–19307 _____.

   **a.** Include partial and complete mastectomy procedures
   **b.** Include radical and modified radical mastectomies
   **c.** Include a mastectomy performed on a male patient
   **d.** All of these statements are true

**10.** [LO 12.1.6] Anesthesia codes for codes in the 10000 integumentary range _____.

   **a.** Are only used for skin and subcutaneous tissue
   **b.** Would not apply to muscle or bone
   **c.** Depend upon the structure or tissue involved
   **d.** Can only be reported by 00300 or 00400

**11.** [LO 12.1.1] Needle aspiration with imaging guidance require code(s) _____.

   **a.** 10021
   **b.** 10022
   **c.** 10022 and a code for radiological supervision and interpretation
   **d.** 10021 and a code for radiological supervision and interpretation

**12.** [LO 12.1.1] Acne surgery is coded as _____.

   **a.** 10060
   **b.** 10140
   **c.** 10040
   **d.** 10160

**13.** [LO 12.1.1] Wound debridement with removal of foreign material at the site of an open fracture, skin and subcutaneous tissues, would be reported as _____.

   **a.** 11012
   **b.** 10120
   **c.** 10120 and 11010
   **d.** 11010

**14.** [LO 12.1.4] Destruction of 11 premalignant lesions of the arms and legs is coded as _____.

   **a.** 17003 ×11
   **b.** 17003 and 17000 (in this order)
   **c.** 17000 and 17003 (in this order)
   **d.** 14000 and 11401 (in this order)

**15.** [LO 12.1.4] Chemosurgery resulting in complete destruction of 16 benign lesions of the face is coded as _____.

   **a.** 17000 and 17003
   **b.** 17000 and 17004
   **c.** 17004
   **d.** 17280

**16.** [LO 12.1.5] Mastectomy on a male patient is coded as _____.

   **a.** 19303
   **b.** 19300
   **c.** 19304
   **d.** 19307

**17.** [LO 12.1.1] Debridement of subcutaneous tissue (including epidermis and dermis) for 40 sq cm is coded as _____.

   **a.** 11042 ×2
   **b.** 11045 ×2
   **c.** 11045, 11042 (in this order)
   **d.** 11042, 11045 (in this order)

**18.** [LO 12.1.2] Simple repair of hand lacerations (right hand 2.0 cm, left hand 0.2 cm) is coded as _____.

   **a.** 12031
   **b.** 12031 ×2
   **c.** 12001 ×2
   **d.** 12001

**19.** [LO 12.1.3] A rotation flap on the abdomen with a primary defect (the excision of a benign lesion) of 1.0 sq cm and a secondary defect (the flap design) of 3.0 sq cm is coded as _____.

   **a.** 14000
   **b.** 14000 and 14001
   **c.** 14001
   **d.** 11400 and 14000

**20.** [LO 12.1.5] Placement of a needle localization wire into a single lesion on the breast preoperatively using radiological image guidance is coded as _____.

   **a.** 19290
   **b.** 19290 and 77031 (in this order)
   **c.** 19290 and 76942 (in this order)
   **d.** 19290 and 19295 (in this order)

## Applying Your Skills

Using your CPT manual, assign the appropriate code(s) for each procedure.

   **1.** [LO 12.1.5] Biopsy of breast not using imaging guidance. _____

   **2.** [LO 12.1.5] Excision of a benign cyst on the left breast of a female. _____

   **3.** [LO 12.1.4] Removal of a gross tumor on the neck using Mohs micrographic technique; first stage, 3 tissue blocks. _____

   **4.** [LO 12.1.3] Excision of a sacral pressure ulcer with skin flap closure. _____

   **5.** [LO 12.1.3] Punch graft for hair transplant; 25 punch grafts. _____

   **6.** [LO 12.1.3] Surgical preparation of an 80 sq cm recipient site with excision of a scar, and the application of a xenograft skin graft, also 80 sq cm, onto the trunk of a male adult patient. _____

   **7.** [LO 12.1.2] Complex repair of 2.0 cm scalp laceration. _____

   **8.** [LO 12.1.2] Secondary closure of a surgical wound dehiscence. _____

   **9.** [LO 12.1.1] Tattooing, using intradermal introduction of insoluble opaque pigments, to correct a 1.2 sq cm color defect of skin of the face. _____

   **10.** [LO 12.1.1] Complicated excision of a pilonidal sinus. _____

## Case Studies

Read each case study. Using your CPT manual, assign the appropriate code(s) to describe each case.

   **1.** [LO 12.1.1] A 17-year-old female, an established patient, came into the office for incision and drainage of a pilonidal cyst. The surgeon deemed this to be a simple case and performed the procedure without complications in the office. _____

   **2.** [LO 12.1.1] A 22-year-old male patient in good health was seen by his family doctor. The patient had developed a severe hematoma after being kicked during a soccer game the week prior. The doctor punctured his hematoma and aspirated the contents. A dressing was placed over the site, and the patient left the office in satisfactory condition. _____

   **3.** [LO 12.1.1] One month postoperatively a 56-year-old male was admitted for a complex incision and drainage of a wound infection and removal of prosthetic mesh material from his abdominal wall. The procedure was accomplished without any complications. _____

**4.** [LO 12.1.1] A 30-year-old patient was seen for the removal of a single 0.8 cm lesion on her right arm. The doctor injected a local anesthetic and removed the lesion by shaving. _____

**5.** [LO 12.1.2] A 12-year-old male was seen in the office following a fall from a bicycle. He incurred several lacerations on his arms and legs, all requiring suture. The patient was complaining of severe pain, but the doctor classified the repair as "simple" and proceeded to repair the wounds. The wounds were noted as follows: right arm 2.0 and 3.2 cm, left arm 5.3 cm, right leg 4.2 cm, and left leg, 1.3 cm and 2.0 cm lacerations. _____

**6.** [LO 12.1.3] A 27-year-old female patient was seen in the office for treatment of deep scarring on her face from the severe acne she had during her teenage years. Her physician determined that dermabrasion would reduce some of the scarring and, with her consent, proceeded to treat her total face. _____

**7.** [LO 12.1.4] A 45-year-old construction worker with long-term sun exposure of his face and arms was seen for removal of the lesions via destruction for the two lesions on his face—1.2 cm and 0.7 cm—and one lesion on his left arm—2.4 cm. _____

## Thinking It Through

Using your critical-thinking skills, answer the following questions.

**1.** [LO 12.1.1] Why would fine needle aspiration be desirable from a patient's point of view versus an incision and drainage procedure?

_____

_____

_____

_____

**2.** [LO 12.1.4] How can a payer validate the medical necessity of a surgical procedure, such as lesion destruction, in which the specimen is "destroyed" and nothing is sent to a pathologist for examination?

_____

_____

_____

_____

**3.** [LO 12.1.1] What are some reasons that patients would have tattooing (CPT code 11920) on their breast?

_____

_____

_____

_____

# MUSCULOSKELETAL SYSTEM

## Learning Outcomes

*After completing this module, students should be able to:*

**12.2.1** Differentiate among musculoskeletal treatment modalities.

**12.2.2** Identify CPT codes that describe general procedures on the musculoskeletal system and procedures on the head, neck, and thorax.

**12.2.3** Describe procedures on the back and flank, spine, and abdomen.

**12.2.4** Determine codes describing procedures on the upper and lower extremities.

**12.2.5** Identify codes that describe the application of casts, strapping, and arthroscopy procedures.

**12.2.6** Code anesthesia services for procedures of the musculoskeletal system.

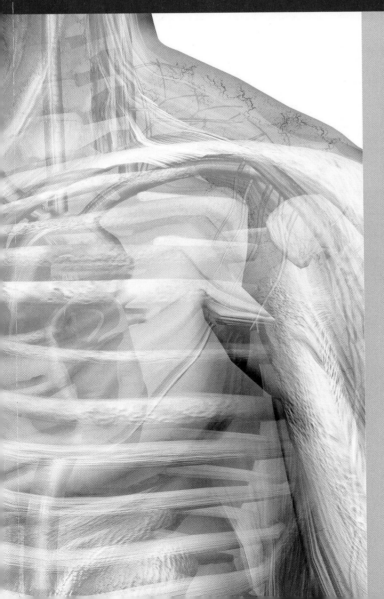

## Introduction

The CPT codes in the 20000 series describe procedures on the musculoskeletal system. These procedure codes are grouped by anatomical regions, including the head, neck, back and flank, spine, abdominal wall, shoulder, upper arm, forearm and wrist, hand and fingers, pelvis and hip joint, femur and knee joint, leg and ankle joint, foot, and toes. Within each anatomical section, subsections of codes describe incision; excision; introduction and removal; repair, revision, and reconstruction; fracture and dislocation repair; arthrodesis; and amputation procedures. Separate sections describe casting/strapping procedures and endoscopic/arthroscopic procedures.

# Key Terms

Define each of the following key terms in the space provided.

1. [LO 12.2.1] Closed fracture _____

_____

2. [LO 12.2.1] Open or compound fracture _____

_____

3. [LO 12.2.1] Comminuted fracture _____

_____

4. [LO 12.2.1] Closed treatment _____

_____

5. [LO 12.2.1] Open treatment _____

_____

6. [LO 12.2.1] Percutaneous skeletal fixation _____

_____

7. [LO 12.2.1] Internal fixation _____

_____

8. [LO 12.2.1] External fixation _____

_____

9. [LO 12.2.1] Traction _____

_____

10. [LO 12.2.1] Manipulation _____

_____

11. [LO 12.2.1] Subcutaneous _____

_____

12. [LO 12.2.2] Penetrating wound _____

_____

13. [LO 12.2.3] Osteotomy _____

_____

14. [LO 12.2.3] Arthrodesis _____

_____

15. [LO 12.2.3] Cervical spine _____

_____

16. [LO 12.2.3] Thoracic spine _____

_____

17. [LO 12.2.3] Lumbar spine _____

_____

18. [LO 12.2.3] Posterior vertebral structure _____

_____

19. [LO 12.2.3] Anterior vertebral structure _____

_____

**20.** [LO 12.2.3] Spinal instrumentation _____
_____

**21.** [LO 12.2.5] Cast _____
_____

**22.** [LO 12.2.5] Splint _____
_____

**23.** [LO 12.2.5] Strapping _____
_____

**24.** [LO 12.2.5] Arthroscopy _____
_____

## Exam Review

Select the letter that best describes the statement or answers the question.

**1.** [LO 12.2.1] Excision of benign and malignant tumors of the face or scalp requires the coder to know _____.
  **a.** The location and size of the tumor
  **b.** Whether the tumor is benign or malignant
  **c.** The method of excision and whether an osteotomy is performed as part of the procedure
  **d.** All of these

**2.** [LO 12.2.1] Soft tissue procedures on the neck and thorax (21501–21899) _____.
  **a.** Exclude excisions of tumors
  **b.** Include excision of tumors
  **c.** Refer to suture and repair of damaged nerves
  **d.** All of these

**3.** [LO 12.2.2] Fusing vertebral bodies and using bone graft material _____.
  **a.** Eliminate the necessity of spinal instrumentation
  **b.** Usually include spinal instrumentation to stabilize vertebral alignment
  **c.** Are seldom performed by surgeons
  **d.** Are performed for traumatic spinal facture only

**4.** [LO 12.2.2] A co-surgeon in a surgical case _____.
  **a.** Is a surgeon of a different specialty from the other surgeon
  **b.** Requires the addition of modifier 80 to the code for the underlying procedure
  **c.** Requires the addition of modifier 62 to the code used by each surgeon for the underlying procedure
  **d.** Both (*a*) and (*c*)

**5.** [LO 12.2.3] Forearm and wrist codes include _____.
  **a.** Reconstruction codes that are based on the treatment type and specific bone
  **b.** Reconstruction codes that are based on the anatomical structure
  **c.** Include the radius, ulna, and carpal bones and joints
  **d.** Both (*b*) and (*c*)

**6.** [LO 12.2.4] Bilateral procedures, such as a decompression fasciotomy of the pelvic compartment, _____.
  **a.** Require the addition of modifier 59 to the code
  **b.** Require the addition of modifier 50 to the code
  **c.** Require modifiers 59 and 50 to the code
  **d.** Require the addition of modifier 58 to the code

**7.** [LO 12.2.3] Incision procedures are _____.

   **a.** Only coded in the Integumentary System section of the CPT manual

   **b.** Not coded in the Integumentary System section of the CPT manual

   **c.** Coded, as appropriate, throughout the Surgery section of the CPT manual

   **d.** Never coded in the Musculoskeletal System section of the CPT manual

**8.** [LO 12.2.5] Once a cast application or strapping procedure or service has been rendered by one physician, _____.

   **a.** Any subsequent physician providing follow-up care for the same patient must be of the same medical specialty

   **b.** Any subsequent care or restorative care by another physician *may not* be reported

   **c.** Any subsequent care or restorative care by another physician *may* be reported

   **d.** The physician classifies the case as definitive and closed

**9.** [LO 12.2.5] E/M service codes are _____.

   **a.** Not reported when a cast or splint is intended to be the definitive treatment of a fracture

   **b.** Reported in addition to the appropriate casting code when a cast or splint is intended to be the definitive treatment of a fracture

   **c.** Not applicable for casting services

   **d.** Only reported for cast removal

**10.** [LO 12.2.4] A diagnostic knee arthroscopy (separate procedure) _____.

   **a.** Is reported only if it is the only procedure performed

   **b.** Is less invasive than an "open" procedure of the knee

   **c.** Can be bundled into a surgical or therapeutic knee arthroscopy procedure

   **d.** All of these

**11.** [LO 12.2.1] Treatment of penetrating wounds that involve surgical exploration and enlargement of the wound but that do not require thoracotomy or laparotomy is in the _____ range of codes.

   **a.** 12020–12021

   **b.** 20101–20102

   **c.** 20100–20103

   **d.** 22010–22015

**12.** [LO 12.2.2] Bone graft codes 20936–20938 are add-on codes that can be used with _____.

   **a.** 22630

   **b.** 22800–22812

   **c.** 22533

   **d.** All of these

**13.** [LO 12.2.1] Tumor excision codes 21930, 21931, 21932, and 21935 are assigned based on the _____.

   **a.** Histology of the tumor

   **b.** Method of resection and histology of the tumor

   **c.** Size of the tumor

   **d.** All of these

**14.** [LO 12.2.3] The appropriate code for incision and drainage of a deep abscess or hematoma in the shoulder area is _____.

   **a.** 10121

   **b.** 23030

   **c.** 23331

   **d.** 10140

**15.** [LO 12.2.4] Arthroscopy, knee, surgical with a medial meniscectomy, is coded as _____.

   **a.** 29868

   **b.** 29880–29882

   **c.** 29880

   **d.** 29881

**16.** [LO 12.2.4]  Arthroscopy, shoulder, distal claviculectomy (Mumford procedure), performed as the only procedure, is coded as _____.

    **a.** 29806

    **b.** 23120

    **c.** 29824

    **d.** 29824-51

**17.** [LO 12.2.3]  Radical resection of a malignant tumor less than 5 cm of the soft tissue area of the shoulder is coded as _____.

    **a.** 23071

    **b.** 23076

    **c.** 23077

    **d.** 23078

**18.** [LO 12.2.1]  Application of multiplane (pins or wires in more than one plane) unilateral, external fixation with stereotactic computer-assisted adjustment, is coded as _____.

    **a.** 20692               **c.** 20696

    **b.** 20692 and 20696 (in this order)    **d.** 20697

**19.** [LO 12.2.1]  Replantation of the thumb (includes distal tip to MP joint), complete amputation, is coded as _____.

    **a.** 20816-52           **c.** 20827

    **b.** 20822              **d.** 20827-52

**20.** [LO 12.2.1]  Aspiration and/or injection of multiple ganglion cysts, any location, is coded as _____.

    **a.** 20600              **c.** 20612-59

    **b.** 20612              **d.** 20612-51

## Applying Your Skills

Using your CPT manual, assign the appropriate code(s) for each procedure.

**1.** [LO 12.2.1]  Exploration of a penetrating wound of the abdomen, no other major structure involved. _____

**2.** [LO 12.2.1]  Deep muscle biopsy. _____

**3.** [LO 12.2.2]  Cartilage graft of the nasal septum. _____

**4.** [LO 12.2.2]  Excision of a 1.2 cm tumor of the soft tissue of the scalp. _____

**5.** [LO 12.2.3]  Superficial biopsy of soft tissue of the back. _____

**6.** [LO 12.2.3]  Incision and drainage of lumbosacral deep abscess of the posterior spine. _____

**7.** [LO 12.2.3]  Partial excision of vertebral body, anterior approach or incision for intrinsic bony lesion, single vertebral segment; cervical. _____

**8.** [LO 12.2.3]  Osteotomy of spine, posterior approach, two vertebral segments; lumbar. _____

**9.** [LO 12.2.4]  Incision and drainage, shoulder area, for infected bursa. _____

**10.** [LO 12.2.4]  Sequestrectomy of the clavicle due to osteomyelitis. _____

## Case Studies

Read each case study. Using your CPT manual, assign the correct code(s) to describe each case.

**1.** [LO 12.2.1]  A 32-year-old male was involved in a bar fight and sustained a stab wound on his right arm. The patient was admitted and taken to the OR for exploration of the surrounding nerves and vessels. The wound was cleansed and closed without complications.

_____

**2.** [LO 12.2.1] A 23-year-old female was seen in radiology for a percutaneous needle muscle biopsy for a suspected malignant growth on her back. Ultrasound guidance was used. Code the procedure and the radiological imaging guidance.

_____

**3.** [LO 12.2.2] A 31-year-old mother of two was seen in an ambulatory surgical center. The patient underwent manipulation of her temporomandibular joint requiring monitored anesthesia care. Code the joint manipulation procedure only.

_____

**4.** [LO 12.2.4] A 24-year-old male avid golfer had an elective rotator cuff repair of his left shoulder following an injury sustained while playing in a golf tournament a week ago.

_____

**5.** [LO 12.2.4] A 12-year-old female was jumping on a trampoline, fell onto the ground, and fractured her clavicle. She was taken to the hospital and admitted for surgery. The surgeon treated her clavicle fracture with an open reduction and internal fixation.

_____

**6.** [LO 12.2.4] An 18-year-old male fell off his street bike and dislocated his hip. He was seen in the emergency room and admitted for surgery. The orthopedic surgeon performed an open treatment of the hip dislocation with internal fixation.

_____

**7.** [LO 12.2.4] A 72-year-old female diabetic was electively scheduled and operated on for a below-knee amputation secondary to a gangrenous leg and foot.

_____

## Thinking It Through

Using your critical-thinking skills, answer the following questions.

**1.** [LO 12.2.4] Arthroscopic procedures have become popular compared to open procedures to accomplish the same surgical results. List several reasons this may be the case.

_____

_____

_____

_____

**2.** [LO 12.2.3] Explain why it is often necessary for two surgeons of different specialties to operate as co-surgeons for spinal procedures. Differentiate the types of spinal procedures that generally require co-surgeons from those that don't.

_____

_____

_____

_____

**3.** [LO 12.2.4] Compare and contrast the terms "open" and "closed" when used to describe fractures with those same terms used to describe the treatment of a fracture. Explain any coding correlation between the type of fracture and the type of treatment.

_____

_____

_____

_____

# RESPIRATORY, CARDIOVASCULAR, HEMIC, AND LYMPHATIC SYSTEMS; MEDIASTINUM AND DIAPHRAGM

## MODULE 12.3

### Learning Outcomes

*After completing this module, students should be able to:*

**12.3.1** Differentiate the surgical procedures performed on the respiratory system.

**12.3.2** Describe the various types of procedures performed on the cardiac system, including coronary artery bypass grafts, repairs of cardiac abnormalities, and procedures on the great vessels.

**12.3.3** Identify CPT codes to report open and endovascular arterial repairs, bypass procedures, angioplasties, shunts, and vascular access procedures.

**12.3.4** Describe procedures on the hemic and lymphatic systems, mediastinum, and diaphragm.

**12.3.5** Code anesthesia services for procedures in the 30000 series of CPT codes

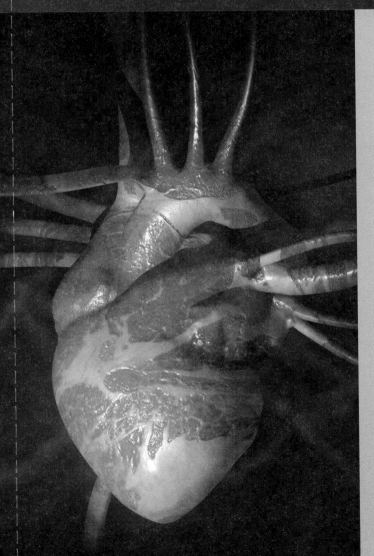

## Introduction

The CPT codes in the 30000 series describe procedures on several organ systems, including the respiratory system, cardiovascular system, and the hemic and lymphatic systems. In addition, these codes describe procedures on anatomical structures located within the mediastinum and on the diaphragm.

The respiratory system includes all structures involved in air exchange from the interior of the nose down through the larynx, trachea, bronchial structures, and lungs. The cardiovascular system includes the heart, pericardium, great vessels, arteries, and veins. Many procedures on the cardiovascular system are described by codes in this series. However, certain nonsurgical procedures on the heart itself, such as percutaneous transluminal coronary angioplasty procedures, are described by codes in the 90000 series. The hemic and lymphatic systems include the bone marrow, spleen, lymph nodes, and lymphatic channels.

# Key Terms

Define each of the following key terms in the space provided.

**1.** [LO 12.3.3] Aneurysm _____

_____

**2.** [LO 12.3.2] Angioplasty _____

**3.** [LO 12.3.1] Bronchi _____

**4.** [LO 12.3.1] Bronchoscopy _____

**5.** [LO 12.3.2] Cardiopulmonary bypass _____

**6.** [LO 12.3.2] Cardiotomy _____

**7.** [LO 12.3.3] Central venous access device _____

**8.** [LO 12.3.1] Diagnostic thoracoscopy _____

**9.** [LO 12.3.3] Embolectomy _____

**10.** [LO 12.3.1] Endoscopy _____

**11.** [LO 12.3.1] Ethmoid sinus _____

**12.** [LO 12.3.3] Extracorporeal membrane oxygenation (ECMO) _____

**13.** [LO 12.3.1] Frontal sinus _____

**14.** [LO 12.3.3] Hemodialysis _____

**15.** [LO 12.3.1] Maxillary sinus _____

**16.** [LO 12.3.4] Mediastinum _____

**17.** [LO 12.3.2] Pericardium _____

**18.** [LO 12.3.1] Pleura _____

**19.** [LO 12.3.2] Shunt _____

_____

**20.** [LO 12.3.1] Sinusotomy _____

_____

**21.** [LO 12.3.1] Sphenoid sinus _____

_____

**22.** [LO 12.3.1] Surgical thoracoscopy _____

_____

**23.** [LO 12.3.3] Thrombectomy _____

_____

**24.** [LO 12.3.1] Trachea _____

_____

**25.** [LO 12.3.1] Turbinate _____

_____

# Exam Review

Select the letter that best describes the statement or answers the question.

1. [LO 12.3.1] The respiratory system includes _____.
   a. The sinuses, larynx, trachea, bronchi, lungs, and pleura but excludes the nose
   b. The sinuses, larynx, trachea, bronchi, lungs, and pleura and includes the nose
   c. Only the lungs
   d. Only the bronchi, lungs, and pleura

2. [LO 12.3.1] Nasal lesions and polyps can be removed by excision or destruction. The primary difference between the two methods is _____.
   a. There is no difference
   b. Both require incisions
   c. In the excision method, tissue could be sent for pathological examination
   d. In the destruction method, tissue could be sent for pathological examination

3. [LO 12.3.1] A surgical sinus endoscopy (codes 31231–31294) _____.
   a. Does not include a diagnostic endoscopy
   b. Includes a diagnostic endoscopy
   c. Includes a sinusotomy when indicated
   d. Both (*b*) and (*c*)

4. [LO 12.3.2] Heart/lung transplantation involves _____.
   a. Cadaver donor organ resection
   b. Backbench work to prepare the donor organ for implantation
   c. Recipient organ transplantation
   d. All of these

5. [LO 12.3.1] Nasal sinuses are _____.
   a. Ethmoid, sphenoid, and maxillary
   b. Frontal, ethmoid, sphenoid, and maxillary
   c. Frontal, posterior, ethmoid, sphenoid, and maxillary
   d. All of the above

**6.** [LO 12.3.1] Nasal endoscopy code 31231 states that the procedure code is for diagnostic, unilateral, or bilateral (separate procedure). If performed bilaterally, the coder would report the code and _____.

    **a.** Add modifier 59

    **b.** Add modifier 51

    **c.** Add modifier 50

    **d.** Would not add modifier 50

**7.** [LO 12.3.1] CPT code 31628 describes bronchoscopy with transbronchial lung biopsy (or biopsies) in a single lobe. If three biopsies are performed on that single lobe, the coder would _____.

    **a.** Report code 31628 × 3, to identify the number of biopsies performed

    **b.** Report code 31628 only once

    **c.** Query the surgeon to obtain more information

    **d.** Use the appropriate add-on code

**8.** [LO 12.3.2] CPT cardiovascular system codes pertain to _____.

    **a.** Nonheart vessels

    **b.** Heart vessels

    **c.** The pericardium and great vessels

    **d.** All of these

**9.** [LO 12.3.2] The pericardium _____.

    **a.** Is the sac that surrounds the heart

    **b.** Can collect too much fluid and decrease the ability of the heart to pump blood

    **c.** Is one of the cardiac vessels

    **d.** Both (*a*) and (*b*)

**10.** [LO 12.3.2] Heart tumors may form _____.

    **a.** Inside the heart (intracardiac)

    **b.** Outside the heart (external tumor)

    **c.** Tumors cannot physiologically grow in or on the heart

    **d.** Both (*a*) and (*b*)

**11.** [LO 12.3.2] CPT code(s) for all aspects of heart transplant, with or without lung allotransplantation, would be _____.

    **a.** 33930–33944

    **b.** 33930–33933

    **c.** 33930–33945

    **d.** 33945

**12.** [LO 12.3.2] A coronary artery bypass graft (CABG) using only a vein graft would be coded as _____.

    **a.** 33510

    **b.** 33510 and 33517 (in this order)

    **c.** 33533

    **d.** 33508

**13.** [LO 12.3.3] The correct code to describe an open repair of a ruptured abdominal aortic aneurysm is _____.

    **a.** 35002

    **b.** 35082

    **c.** 35022

    **d.** 35013

**14.** [LO 12.3.4] A diagnostic laparoscopy resulted in a surgical laparoscopic splenectomy. The correct code(s) to describe these procedures would be _____.

    **a.** 38100

    **b.** 38100 and 38102 (in this order)

    **c.** 49320 and 38120 (in this order)

    **d.** 38120

    

**15.** [LO 12.3.4]  The correct code for bone marrow aspiration is _____.

    **a.** 38220
    **b.** 38230
    **c.** 38205
    **d.** 38212

**16.** [LO 12.3.4]  Open, biopsy of superficial lymph nodes is coded as _____.

    **a.** 38500 and 38780 (in this order)
    **b.** 38510
    **c.** 38542
    **d.** 38500

**17.** [LO 12.3.4]  Repair of an acute ruptured diaphragmatic hernia in an adult patient is coded as _____.

    **a.** 43281
    **b.** 39503
    **c.** 39501
    **d.** 39540

**18.** [LO 12.3.1]  A bilobectomy is coded as _____.

    **a.** 32480
    **b.** 32440
    **c.** 32482
    **d.** 32320

**19.** [LO 12.3.1]  A diagnostic thoracoscopy revealed a mass in the mediastinal space. The surgeon proceeded to obtain a biopsy of the mass. These procedures are coded as _____.

    **a.** 32606
    **b.** 32601 and 32606 (in this order)
    **c.** 32662
    **d.** 32606 and 32662

**20.** [LO 12.3.2]  Insertion of a permanent pacemaker with transvenous electrode(s) into the right atrium and ventricle is coded as _____.

    **a.** 33212
    **b.** 33206 and 33207
    **c.** 33211
    **d.** 33208

## Applying Your Skills

Using your CPT manual, assign the appropriate code(s) to each procedure.

  **1.** [LO 12.3.2]  Resection of an external tumor on the heart. _____

  **2.** [LO 12.3.2]  Pericardiotomy for removal of foreign body. _____

  **3.** [LO 12.3.2]  Conversion from single-chamber pacemaker system to dual-chamber system. _____

  **4.** [LO 12.3.2]  Revision of skin pocket for cardioverter-defibrillator. _____

  **5.** [LO 12.3.3]  Embolectomy of brachial artery, without catheter, by arm incision. _____

  **6.** [LO 12.3.3]  Endovascular repair infrarenal abdominal aortic dissection using modular bifurcated prosthesis (one docking limb). _____

  **7.** [LO 12.3.3]  Valvuloplasty of the femoral vein. _____

  **8.** [LO 12.3.2]  Pericardiocentesis, initial. _____

  **9.** [LO 12.3.2]  Removal and reinsertion of a single-chamber pacing cardioverter-defibrillator system (pulse generator and electrodes) by thoracotomy. _____

  **10.** [LO 12.3.2]  Initial implantation of patient-activated cardiac event recorder. _____

# Case Studies

Read each case study. Using your CPT manual, assign the correct code(s) to describe each case.

**1.** [LO 12.3.2] A 62-year-old male was admitted for a triple-bypass elective CABG. One arterial graft and two venous grafts were used. There were no complications during the procedure.

_____

**2.** [LO 12.3.3] A 21-year-old female trauma patient was one of the passengers involved in a three-car accident with one of the cars rolling over. The patient's neck was severely lacerated, and she was taken to the OR for a direct repair of her carotid artery. Code the repair.

_____

**3.** [LO 12.3.3] An 84-year-old patient was admitted for elective surgery. The nurse was not able to start an IV. The physician was requested to perform a venipuncture cutdown to establish intravenous access for fluids and medication. Code the cutdown.

_____

**4.** [LO 12.3.3] A 2-day-old female newborn required a complete exchange transfusion. The physician calculated the exact blood volume needed. The patient's blood was removed and replaced simultaneously without complication. Code the exchange transfusion.

_____

**5.** [LO 12.3.1] A 27-year-old male was comatose following an overdose of prescription pain medication. At the time of his arrival via ambulance, he was intubated via endotracheal tube and placed on a ventilator. Several days later he was taken to the OR for a tracheostomy and insertion of a tracheostomy tube. Report the tracheostomy.

_____

**6.** [LO 12.3.1] Two days later, this same patient had his indwelling tracheotomy tube replaced with a new one. Report the tube change.

_____

**7.** [LO 12.3.1] A 45-year-old male was scheduled for an elective diagnostic flexible fiberoptic laryngoscopy with possible removal of the lesion. During the procedure, the physician removed a lesion. Code the laryngoscopy.

_____

**8.** [LO 12.3.1] A 50-year-old female had elective surgery for removal of a malignant tracheal tumor. Via a thoracic approach to access the mass, the trachea was incised and the mass resected. The wound was closed and sutured in layers. Pathological interpretation of the specimen confirmed the pre- and postoperative diagnoses of cancer.

_____

**9.** [LO 12.3.1] A 67-year-old male smoker with a 45-year history of smoking was admitted for an elective thoracotomy and lung biopsy of a lung nodule. No complications occurred.

_____

**10.** [LO 12.3.1] A 35-year-old female was electively admitted for a percutaneous needle biopsy of the mediastinum. The patient was discharged home the same day.

_____

# Thinking It Through

Using your critical-thinking skills, answer the following questions.

1. [LO 12.3.2] Compare and contrast PTCA and CABG procedures.

   _____

   _____

   _____

   _____

2. [LO 12.3.1] According to the CPT manual, surgical endoscopic procedures, e.g., bronchoscopies, thoracoscopies, etc., always include diagnostic endoscopic procedures. Why do you think the rule is set up this way?

   _____

   _____

   _____

   _____

3. [LO 12.3.3] What is the first thing the coder must determine before selecting the code for a percutaneous transluminal angioplasty procedure?

   _____

   _____

   _____

   _____

4. [LO 12.3.2] Describe how coronary artery bypass graft (CABG) procedures are reported using CPT codes.

   _____

   _____

   _____

   _____

5. [LO 12.3.1] Compare and contrast CPT codes 32440, 32480, 32482, and 32484.

   _____

   _____

   _____

   _____

# MODULE

# 12.4 DIGESTIVE SYSTEM

## Learning Outcomes

*After completing this module, students should be able to:*

**12.4.1** Identify procedures on the digestive system from the lips to the throat.

**12.4.2** Describe procedures on the digestive tract from the esophagus to the anus.

**12.4.3** Identify procedures on organ systems attached to the gastrointestinal tract.

**12.4.4** Code anesthesia for procedures in the 40000 series.

## Introduction

The CPT codes in the 40000 series include procedures on the entire digestive system. The gastrointestinal (GI) tract is an irregular tubular structure that begins at the lips and continues uninterrupted until it ends at the anus. The digestive system consists of the GI tract and additional organs and anatomical structures that attach to the GI tract. The CPT codes describing procedures on the digestive system are divided according to the anatomical section of the GI tract or associated organs. The CPT codes within each anatomical division are further subdivided according to the type of procedure, such as incision, excision, repair, endoscopy, or laparoscopy.

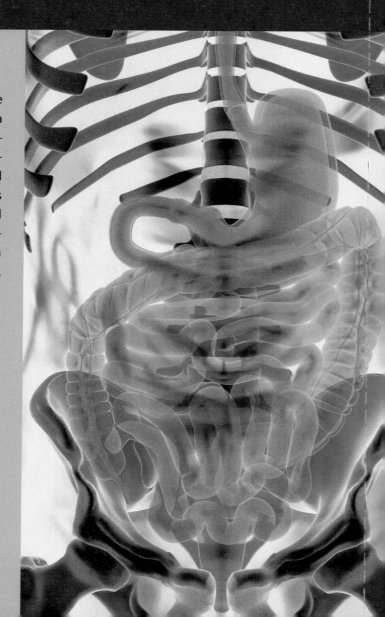

# Key Terms

Define each of the following key terms in the space provided.

**1.** [LO 12.4.2]  Appendix _____

_____

**2.** [LO 12.4.3]  Backbench work _____

_____

**3.** [LO 12.4.2]  Colonoscopy _____

_____

**4.** [LO 12.4.2]  Endoscopic retrograde cholangiopancreatography (ERCP) _____

_____

**5.** [LO 12.4.2]  Endoscopy _____

_____

**6.** [LO 12.4.2]  Fistula _____

_____

**7.** [LO 12.4.2]  Gastrointestinal _____

_____

**8.** [LO 12.4.2]  Intestines _____

_____

**9.** [LO 12.4.2]  Laparoscopy _____

_____

**10.** [LO 12.4.2]  Proctectomy _____

_____

# Exam Review

Select the letter that best describes the statement or answers the question.

**1.** [LO 12.4.1]  The gastrointestinal system begins _____.
   **a.** With the esophagus and continues to the anus
   **b.** With the stomach and continues to the anus
   **c.** With the lips and continues to the anus
   **d.** With colon loops and continues to the anus

**2.** [LO 12.4.1]  Incision, excision, and repair procedures can be coded using _____.
   **a.** Only Integumentary System section codes
   **b.** Only Evaluation and Management (E/M) section codes if the procedure is done in the doctor's office
   **c.** Only Digestive System section codes
   **d.** Any appropriate system or section codes for procedures performed in various settings

**3.** [LO 12.4.1]  Procedures on the lips and surrounding skin are described by codes from the _____.
   **a.** Digestive System section only
   **b.** Digestive and Integumentary System sections
   **c.** Integumentary System section only
   **d.** Using unlisted procedure code 40799

**4.** [LO 12.4.2]  Esophagotomies can be coded _____.

    **a.** Using codes 43020 and 43045

    **b.** To include removing a foreign body

    **c.** Designating either a cervical approach or thoracic approach

    **d.** All of the above

**5.** [LO 12.4.2]  When an appendectomy is performed as an incidental procedure, it is _____.

    **a.** Not coded

    **b.** Coded as 44955

    **c.** Coded as 44950 without a modifier

    **d.** Coded as 44950 with modifier 52 if it is necessary to report the procedure

**6.** [LO 12.4.2]  The main difference between a laparoscopic appendectomy and an appendectomy via a surgical incision is _____.

    **a.** There is no difference

    **b.** No change in physician's approach because "surgery is surgery" and laparoscopic procedures require small incisions

    **c.** The surgeon's approach

    **d.** The anesthesia used

**7.** [LO 12.4.2]  The acronym ERCP stands for _____.

    **a.** Enterolysis retrograde cholangiopancreatography

    **b.** Esophagectomy retrograde cholangiopancreatography

    **c.** Exeresis retrograde cholangiopancreatography

    **d.** Endoscopic retrograde cholangiopancreatography

**8.** [LO 12.4.3]  Liver transplantation codes (47133–47147) include the following component(s) of physician work: _____.

    **a.** Living donor hepatectomy

    **b.** Cadaver donor hepatectomy

    **c.** Backbench work and recipient liver allotransplantation

    **d.** All of the above

**9.** [LO 12.4.3]  The biliary tract includes the _____.

    **a.** Cystic duct

    **b.** Carina cavernosa

    **c.** Common bile duct and extrahepatic portion of the hepatic duct

    **d.** Both (*a*) and (*c*)

**10.** [LO 12.4.3]  Abdomen, peritoneum, and omentum codes (49000–49999) _____.

    **a.** Exclude the peritoneum and omentum if laparoscopically explored

    **b.** Exclude "open" approaches

    **c.** Exclude percutaneous approaches

    **d.** Include laparoscopic and open approaches

**11.** [LO 12.4.3]  A hepatotomy for percutaneous drainage of a cyst, one stage, without radiological supervision and interpretation, is coded as _____.

    **a.** 47010

    **b.** 75989

    **c.** 47011 and 75989

    **d.** 47011

**12.** [LO 12.4.3]  Laparoscopic, cryosurgical ablation of one or more liver tumors is coded as _____.

    **a.** 47370

    **b.** 47370 and 47371 (in this order)

    **c.** 47371 and 76940 (in this order)

    **d.** 47371

**13.** [LO 12.4.2] A diagnostic ERCP with moderate sedation by the same physician and radiological supervision and interpretation is reported with code(s) _____.

**a.** 43260 and 99143
**b.** 43260
**c.** 43260 and 74328
**d.** 43260, 74328, and 99143

**14.** [LO 12.4.2] Diagnostic flexible esophagoscopy with multiple biopsies is coded as _____.

**a.** 43200 and 43202
**b.** 43200 and 99143
**c.** 43202 and 99143
**d.** 43202

**15.** [LO 12.4.1] CPT code 41800 describes the procedure _____.

**a.** Abscess drainage of a tooth
**b.** Drainage of the tooth socket, not the tooth itself
**c.** Both (*a*) and (*b*)
**d.** Neither (*a*) nor (*b*)

**16.** [LO 12.4.1] Cheiloplasty, full thickness, half vertical height, is coded as _____.

**a.** 40650 and 40652
**b.** 40650 and 40654
**c.** 40652
**d.** 40654

**17.** [LO 12.4.1] Excision of a lesion of the vestibule of mouth without repair is coded as _____.

**a.** 40818
**b.** 40810
**c.** 40820
**d.** 40804

**18.** [LO 12.4.1] Gingivectomy is coded as _____.

**a.** 41874
**b.** 41870
**c.** 41820 and 41870 (in this order)
**d.** 41820

**19.** [LO 12.4.1] Glossectomy, composite procedure with resection of floor of mouth and mandibular resection, without radical neck dissection, is coded as _____.

**a.** 41140
**b.** 41150
**c.** 41120 and 41140 (in this order)
**d.** 41120 and 41150 (in this order)

**20.** [LO 12.4.1] Pharyngoplasty is coded as _____.

**a.** 42900
**b.** 42950
**c.** 42953
**d.** 42900 and 42953

## Applying Your Skills

Using your CPT manual, assign the appropriate code(s) for each procedure.

**1.** [LO 12.4.2] Excision of esophageal lesion, cervical approach, with primary repair. _____

**2.** [LO 12.4.2] Near total esophagectomy with thoracotomy. _____

**3.** [LO 12.4.2]  Esophagoscopy with removal of foreign body. _____

**4.** [LO 12.4.2]  Laparoscopy, surgical, repair of paraesophageal hernia with mesh implantation. _____

**5.** [LO 12.4.2]  Retrograde balloon dilation of esophagus, with radiological supervision and interpretation. _____

**6.** [LO 12.4.2]  Biopsy of stomach, by laparotomy. _____

**7.** [LO 12.4.2]  Laparoscopic placement of gastric band. _____

**8.** [LO 12.4.3]  Wedge biopsy of liver. _____

**9.** [LO 12.4.3]  Hepatectomy, partial lobectomy of liver. _____

**10.** [LO 12.4.3]  Cryosurgical laparoscopic ablation of liver tumor. _____

## Case Studies

Read each case study. Using your CPT manual, assign the appropriate code(s) to describe each case.

**1.** [LO 12.4.3]  A 45-year-old male with a gunshot wound to the abdomen was brought to the emergency room by ambulance and taken to surgery for an open exploratory laparotomy of the retroperitoneal area.

_____

**2.** [LO 12.4.3]  The same patient as above, now three days postop, developed a peritoneal abscess requiring a return to the operating room for drainage of the abscess via an open surgical approach.

_____

**3.** [LO 12.4.2]  A 29-year-old female with acute ruptured appendicitis was seen in the doctor's office and subsequently admitted and taken to surgery for removal of the appendix via an abdominal incision.

_____

**4.** [LO 12.4.2]  A 56-year-old male had been suffering with hemorrhoids for several years. He finally sought medical intervention and was taken to surgery for a complex removal of internal and external hemorrhoids involving two columns.

_____

**5.** [LO 12.4.2]  A 31-year-old male weighing 360 lb was admitted for a laparoscopic gastric bypass with small intestine reconstruction to limit absorption.

_____

**6.** [LO 12.4.2]  A 34-year-old female was admitted for an open surgical repair of a bleeding stomach ulcer using a suture repair technique.

_____

**7.** [LO 12.4.1]  A 14-year-old female with a history of severe, chronic tonsillitis was taken to surgery for an elective tonsillectomy.

_____

## Thinking It Through

Using your critical-thinking skills, answer the following questions.

**1.** [LO 12.4.2]  Explain the difference between an exploratory abdominal laparotomy and an exploratory abdominal laparoscopy.

_____

_____

_____

_____

**2.** [LO 12.4.2] In cases where the colon is examined, what is the determining factor whether to use a code from the colonoscopy, proctosigmoidoscopy, or sigmoidoscopy range of codes?

_____

_____

_____

_____

**3.** [LO 12.4.2] According to the CPT manual, placement of a nasogastric tube (CPT code 43752) is located in the alphabetic index under "Placement." However, when the code is verified in the Digestive System subsection of the manual, it is under the subheading entitled "Introduction." What should coders do to improve their coding accuracy when differences between the alphabetic index and the actual code location within the section of the CPT manual occur?

_____

_____

_____

_____

# 12.5

# URINARY SYSTEM, MALE AND FEMALE GENITAL SYSTEMS, AND MATERNITY CARE AND DELIVERY

## Learning Outcomes

*After completing this module, students should be able to:*

**12.5.1** Report codes for procedures on the urinary system.

**12.5.2** Describe codes for procedures on the male genital system.

**12.5.3** Describe codes for procedures on the female genital system.

**12.5.4** Explain codes used to report maternity care services.

**12.5.5** Select anesthesia codes for procedures in the 50000 series.

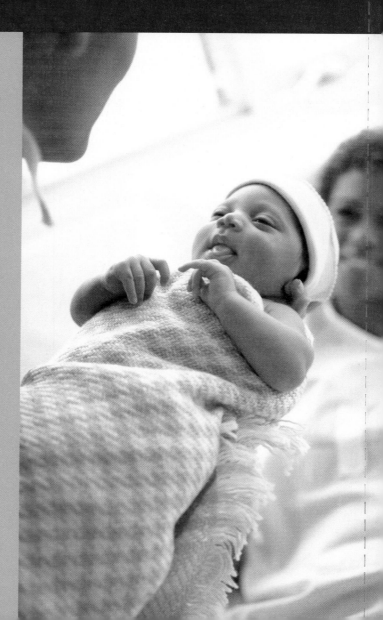

## Introduction

The CPT codes in the 50000 series can are divided into four separate sections. The first section of codes describes procedures on the urinary system. Most of these are the same or very similar in both male and female patients, such as procedures on the kidneys, ureters, bladder, and transurethral cystoscopic procedures. Some procedures, however, are unique to one gender or the other, such as the transurethral resection of the prostate (TURP) or the transurethral radiofrequency microremodeling of urethra in women for stress incontinence.

The second section describes procedures that are unique to the male genital system, while the third describes procedures on the female genital system. The fourth section describes maternity care and delivery services, including prenatal care, vaginal and cesarean deliveries, delivery after previous cesarean delivery, and postpartum care.

# Key Terms

Define each of the following key terms in the space provided.

**1.** [LO 12.5.1] Allotransplantation _____

_____

**2.** [LO 12.5.4] Antepartum care _____

**3.** [LO 12.5.3] Bartholin gland _____

**4.** [LO 12.5.1] Bladder _____

_____

**5.** [LO 12.5.3] Cervix _____

_____

**6.** [LO 12.5.4] Cesarean section _____

_____

**7.** [LO 12.5.3] Colposcopy _____

_____

**8.** [LO 12.5.3] Cystocele _____

_____

**9.** [LO 12.5.3] Endometrium _____

_____

**10.** [LO 12.5.3] Enterocele _____

**11.** [LO 12.5.2] Epididymis _____

**12.** [LO 12.5.2] Epispadias _____

**13.** [LO 12.5.2] Hypospadias _____

_____

**14.** [LO 12.5.1] Kidney _____

_____

**15.** [LO 12.5.3] Myometrium _____

_____

**16.** [LO 12.5.2] Orchiopexy _____

_____

**17.** [LO 12.5.4] Postpartum care _____

_____

**18.** [LO 12.5.2] Prostate _____

_____

**19.** [LO 12.5.3] Rectocele _____

_____

**20.** [LO 12.5.1] Renal calculus _____

_____

**21.** [LO 12.5.2] Seminal vesicle _____

_____

**22.** [LO 12.5.2] Testis or testicle _____

_____

**23.** [LO 12.5.2] Tunica vaginalis _____

_____

**24.** [LO 12.5.1] Ureter _____

_____

**25.** [LO 12.5.1] Urethra _____

_____

**26.** [LO 12.5.3] Vagina _____

_____

**27.** [LO 12.5.4] Vaginal delivery _____

_____

**28.** [LO 12.5.2] Vas deferens (spermatic cord) _____

_____

**29.** [LO 12.5.4] VBAC _____

_____

**30.** [LO 12.5.3] Vulva _____

_____

## Exam Review

Select the letter that best describes the statement or answers the question.

**1.** [LO 12.5.1] The urinary system consists of the _____.
   **a.** Kidney and the bladder
   **b.** Kidneys, ureters, and the bladder
   **c.** Kidneys, ureters, urethra, and the bladder
   **d.** Kidneys and interior tubular structures

**2.** [LO 12.5.1] The primary difference between the male and female urinary systems involves _____.
   **a.** There are no significant differences between these systems
   **b.** The urethral structures
   **c.** Internal differences related to the kidneys
   **d.** The urethra and surrounding structures between the outlet of the bladder and the meatus

**3.** [LO 12.5.1] Incision procedures on the kidney include _____.
   **a.** Drainage of abscess
   **b.** Removal of kidney stones
   **c.** Placement of nephrostomy tube
   **d.** All of these

**4.** [LO 12.5.1] Kidney transplant codes include _____.

   **a.** Living donors

   **b.** Cadaver donors

   **c.** Nephrectomy, backbench work on the donor organ and organ transplantation

   **d.** All of these

**5.** [LO 12.5.1] Urethral and ureteral stents are functionally used _____.

   **a.** To allow urine to drain from the kidney

   **b.** As grafts for the anatomical structures within the urinary system

   **c.** To keep the urethra and ureter patent, allowing urine to drain from the kidney into the bladder or from the bladder to the external environment.

   **d.** Both (*b*) and (*c*)

**6.** [LO 12.5.3] CPT codes 57200–57355 describe repair codes _____.

   **a.** Based on the underlying defect

   **b.** Include cystocele, rectocele, enterocele, and other pelvic floor defects

   **c.** Are differentiated by vaginal and abdominal approaches

   **d.** All of these

**7.** [LO 12.5.3] CPT code 58800 contains the term "unilateral or bilateral." This indicates to the coder that _____.

   **a.** The code must be reported twice for bilateral procedures

   **b.** The code is reported only once for bilateral procedures

   **c.** Modifier 50 must be added for bilateral procedures

   **d.** All of these

**8.** [LO 12.5.3] CPT code 58720 is a salpingo-oophorectomy that is also noted to be a "separate procedure." This indicates to the coder that _____.

   **a.** This code is appropriate if it is the only procedure performed

   **b.** This code can only be used if it is part of another major procedure

   **c.** This code cannot be used if it is performed as part of another major procedure

   **d.** Both (*a*) and (*c*)

**9.** [LO 12.5.4] When reporting maternity care and delivery services, the coder must _____.

   **a.** Include antepartum care codes

   **b.** Utilize codes reflecting delivery service only

   **c.** Include appropriate postpartum codes

   **d.** Know if the service involved antepartum care, delivery, and postpartum care

**10.** [LO 12.5.4] Delivery of patients who have had a previous cesarean delivery and now present with the expectation of a vaginal delivery are coded _____.

   **a.** As a "vaginal delivery" only

   **b.** Based on whether the attempted vaginal birth is successful or not

   **c.** As an "obstetrical" package

   **d.** The same as any other delivery

**11.** [LO 12.5.4] Use code(s) _____ for an unsuccessful VBAC attempt followed by a cesarean delivery.

   **a.** 59514

   **b.** 59514 and 59515

   **c.** 59610

   **d.** 59618–59622 as appropriate

**12.** [LO 12.5.4] Postpartum care only after cesarean delivery is coded as _____.
 a. 59515
 b. 59430
 c. 59622
 d. 59410

**13.** [LO 12.5.4] Biopsy of three lesions of the perineum is coded as _____.
 a. 56605 ×3
 b. 56605 and 56606
 c. 56605 and 56606-51
 d. 56605 and 56606 ×2

**14.** [LO 12.5.3] Colpoperineorrhaphy (nonobstetrical) is coded as _____.
 a. 57240
 b. 57200
 c. 57210
 d. 57260

**15.** [LO 12.5.2] Radical amputation of penis is coded as _____.
 a. 54120
 b. 54130
 c. 54125
 d. 54125-59

**16.** [LO 12.5.4] Bilateral vasotomy is coded as _____.
 a. 55400
 b. 55300-50
 c. 55300
 d. 55250

**17.** [LO 12.5.3] Laparoscopic follicle puncture for oocyte retrieval is coded as _____.
 a. 58970
 b. 58970 and 76948 (in this order)
 c. 58974
 d. 58976

**18.** [LO 12.5.4] Amniocentesis for therapeutic amniotic fluid reduction is coded as _____.
 a. 59000 and 76946 (in this order)
 b. 59000 and 59001 (in this order)
 c. 59001 and 76946
 d. 59001

**19.** [LO 12.5.4] Surgical treatment of ectopic pregnancy, ovarian, without salpingectomy, is coded as _____.
 a. 59150
 b. 59120
 c. 59121
 d. 59151

**20.** [LO 12.5.4] Surgical repair of a ruptured uterus (obstetrical) is coded as _____.
 a. 58520
 b. 58540
 c. 58579
 d. 59350

# Applying Your Skills

Using your CPT manual, assign the appropriate code(s) for each procedure.

1. [LO 12.5.2] Chemical destruction of two lesions on a penis. _____

2. [LO 12.5.2] Circumcision of a baby 29 days old. _____

3. [LO 12.5.2] Bilateral orchiopexy, inguinal approach, with hernia repair. _____

4. [LO 12.5.2] Bilateral vasectomy of a 27-year-old male. _____

5. [LO 12.5.3] Hymenotomy via a simple incision. _____

6. [LO 12.5.3] Excision of a Bartholin cyst. _____

7. [LO 12.5.3] Incision and drainage of a postpartum vaginal hematoma. _____

8. [LO 12.5.3] Biopsy of a single cyst, vaginal mucosa, extensive. _____

9. [LO 12.5.3] Irrigation and flushing of vagina for treatment of a parasitic disease. _____

10. [LO 12.5.4] Postpartum care only following a normal, vaginal delivery. _____

# Case Studies

Reach each case study. Using your CPT manual, assign the appropriate code(s) to describe each case.

1. [LO 12.5.1] A 42-year-old male was taken to surgery for exploration and drainage of a perirenal abscess. Drainage tubes were placed and sutured. The wound was packed with gauze and the muscles were sutured. The skin and subcutaneous tissue were left open.

   _____

2. [LO 12.5.1] A 35-year-old female with a congenital kidney malformation presented with symptomatic pain and confirmed kidney stones. She was taken to surgery for a nephrolithotomy with removal of the stones. Intraoperatively, the surgeon experienced more difficulty with the procedure due to the patient's kidney malformation but ultimately concluded the case without any complications.

   _____

3. [LO 12.5.1] After a vehicle accident, a 49-year-old male trauma patient was officially declared brain dead. Plans were made to take the patient to the OR for organ harvesting in accordance with the patient's predetermined wishes and the family's consent. The surgeon removed both kidneys and packed them for transport. Code the organ harvesting procedure and then continue with the case listed below.

   _____

4. [LO 12.5.1] In the next county, a 21-year-old male with kidney failure was awaiting donor kidneys. The patient was already hospitalized and was now prepared for surgery. The patient was taken to the OR for removal of his kidneys and a renal allotransplantation. Code the recipient procedure(s).

   _____

5. [LO 12.5.2] A 56-year-old male was taken to surgery for an incisional biopsy of the prostate. The specimen was sent to the lab for pathological examination. Code the surgical procedure only.

   _____

6. [LO 12.5.3] An 82-year-old female was electively admitted and taken to surgery for repair of a vaginal prolapse. The surgeon performed a colpopexy via an abdominal incision. There were no complications intraoperatively.

   _____

7. [LO 12.5.3] A 41-year-old female was admitted for laparoscopic vaginal hysterectomy and salpingo-oophorectomy. Uterine weight was noted to be 282 g. The procedure was carried out without complications.

   _____

# Thinking It Through

Using your critical-thinking skills, answer the following questions.

1. [LO 12.5.4]  If an obstetrician performs a cesarean delivery, is this enough information to accurately code the procedure?

   _____

   _____

   _____

   _____

2. [LO 12.5.1]  What is the difference between cadaver and living organ donation/harvesting?

   _____

   _____

   _____

   _____

3. [LO 12.5.1]  How can coders improve their coding accuracy and avoid making "reading" errors on medical terms that are very similar, e.g., ureteral and urethral?

   _____

   _____

   _____

   _____

# ENDOCRINE, NERVOUS, OCULAR, AND AUDITORY SYSTEMS

## Learning Outcomes

*After completing this module, students should be able to:*

**12.6.1** Differentiate among procedures on the endocrine system.

**12.6.2** Contrast procedures on the skull, meninges, and brain.

**12.6.3** Explain procedures involving the spine and spinal cord.

**12.6.4** Identify procedures on extracranial nerves, peripheral nerves, and the autonomic nervous system.

**12.6.5** Describe the major anatomical structures of the eye and surgical procedures performed on those structures.

**12.6.6** Explain the major procedures performed on the auditory system.

**12.6.7** Code anesthesia services for procedures in the 60000 series.

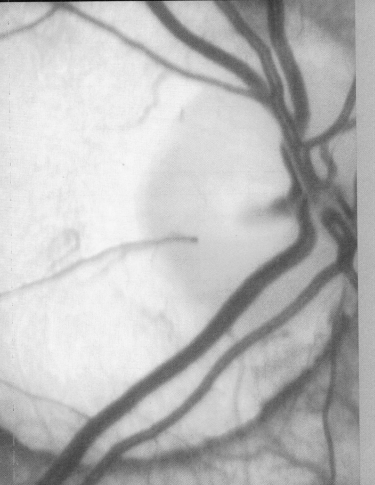

## Introduction

The CPT codes in the 60000 series describe procedures on the endocrine system; the nervous system, including the brain, spine and spinal cord, extracranial nerves, peripheral nerves, and the auto nervous system; the eye and other ocular structures; and the auditory system. Additionally, one code describes the use of an operating microscope. The codes describing procedures on the endocrine system are identified with code numbers in the 60000 series, but are located at the end of the 50000 code series in the CPT manual.

# Key Terms

Define each of the following key terms in the space provided.

**1.** [LO 12.6.1] Adrenal gland _____

_____

**2.** [LO 12.6.2] Anterior cranial fossa _____

_____

**3.** [LO 12.6.2] Arteriovenous malformation _____

_____

**4.** [LO 12.6.1] Carotid body _____

_____

**5.** [LO 12.6.2] Craniectomy _____

_____

**6.** [LO 12.6.2] Cranioplasty _____

_____

**7.** [LO 12.6.2] Craniotomy _____

_____

**8.** [LO 12.6.3] Epidural _____

_____

**9.** [LO 12.6.2] Extracranial artery _____

_____

**10.** [LO 12.6.2] Frontal bone _____

_____

**11.** [LO 12.6.1] Gonad _____

_____

**12.** [LO 12.6.2] Infratentorial _____

_____

**13.** [LO 12.6.2] Intracranial artery _____

_____

**14.** [LO 12.6.3] Intrathecal _____

_____

**15.** [LO 12.6.2] Meninges _____

_____

**16.** [LO 12.6.2] Middle cranial fossa _____

_____

**17.** [LO 12.6.2] Occipital bones _____

_____

**18.** [LO 12.6.1] Pancreas _____

_____

**19.** [LO 12.6.1] Parathyroid gland _____

_____

**20.** [LO 12.6.2] Parietal bone _____

_____

**21.** [LO 12.6.1] Pineal gland _____

_____

**22.** [LO 12.6.1] Pituitary gland _____

_____

**23.** [LO 12.6.2] Posterior cranial fossa _____

_____

**24.** [LO 12.6.2] Supratentorial _____

_____

**25.** [LO 12.6.2] Temporal bone _____

_____

**26.** [LO 12.6.1] Thymus _____

_____

**27.** [LO 12.6.1] Thyroid _____

_____

## Exam Review

Select the answer that best describes the statement or answers the question.

**1.** [LO 12.6.1] CPT code 60512, parathyroid autotransplantation, reports _____.

   **a.** The reimplantation of donor parathyroid glands

   **b.** The reimplantation of parathyroid glands from the patient's own body

   **c.** The initial implantation of parathyroid glands from the patient's own body

   **d.** None of these

**2.** [LO 12.6.1] The following applies to procedures on male and female gonads (testes and ovaries), which are part of the endocrine system:

   **a.** They are coded by using any appropriate code from the range 60000–60699.

   **b.** They are coded as "unlisted" codes 60659 or 60699 since no other code in the range specifically names them.

   **c.** They are actually coded in the reproductive endocrine system for male and female genital systems, not in 60000–60699.

   **d.** None of these.

**3.** [LO 12.6.2] Twist drills, burr drills, and trephines for skull, meninges, and brain procedures _____.

   **a.** Are manual and electric tools used by neurosurgeons intraoperatively

   **b.** Are types of equipment used only by surgery techs to assist the operating neurosurgeon during the case

   **c.** Have been replaced by "stereotactic" equipment

   **d.** None of these

**4.** [LO 12.6.2] Craniotomy codes such as 61556, 61546, and/or 61537 _____.

   **a.** Are not used for "excision" procedures because craniectomy codes cover all excision procedures

   **b.** Could be classified as an "excision" procedure even though the suffix -otomy means "to make an incision into or cut into" while the suffix -ectomy means "surgical removal"

   **c.** Are performed for the treatment of arteriovenous malformations

   **d.** None of these

**5.** [LO 12.6.4] According to the CPT manual, codes 64702–64727 involve _____.

    **a.** Nerve repair and restoration

    **b.** Exploring and freeing nerves, but not nerve transposition

    **c.** Decompression of intact nerves

    **d.** Neuroplasty including external neurolysis and/or transposition

**6.** [LO 12.6.5] With respect to eyes _____.

    **a.** Keratoplasty and cryotherapy codes are synonymous with each other

    **b.** Keratoplasty codes relate to transplant operations of the cornea, and cryotherapy involves the use of a freezing probe on the corneal defect to destroy it

    **c.** Keratoplasty and cryotherapy reflect two entirely different therapies

    **d.** Both (*b*) and (*c*)

**7.** [LO 12.6.4] Neurostimulators are placed _____.

    **a.** Via open surgical exposure of the area

    **b.** Percutaneously

    **c.** Both (*a*) and (*b*)

    **d.** None of these

**8.** [LO 12.6.5] The medical term "exenteration" as in CPT code 65110 _____.

    **a.** Means the same as "evisceration"

    **b.** Refers to removal of the inner organs

    **c.** Is the exact opposite of prosthetic appendage modification

    **d.** Both (*a*) and (*b*)

**9.** [LO 12.6.5] According to the CPT manual, "secondary implant(s) procedures" occur either inside or outside the muscular cone of the eye. These implants can be _____.

    **a.** Orbital implants, inside the muscular cone, and ocular implants, outside the muscular cone

    **b.** Ocular implants, inside the muscular cone, and orbital implants, outside the muscular cone

    **c.** Eviscerated and synthetic scleral shell material made for eye use only

    **d.** None of these

**10.** [LO 12.6.6] Bilateral removal of impacted cerumen (ear wax) is reported as _____.

    **a.** 69210-50

    **b.** 69210

    **c.** 69200

    **d.** None of these

**11.** [LO 12.6.6] The correct code for drainage of an external auditory canal abscess is _____.

    **a.** 69000

    **b.** 69005

    **c.** 69220

    **d.** 69020

**12.** [LO 12.6.5] Repair of a nonperforating corneal laceration without removal of foreign body is coded as _____.

    **a.** 65220

    **b.** 65275

    **c.** 65222

    **d.** None of these

**13.** [LO 12.6.5] Corneal biopsy is coded as _____.

    **a.** 65430

    **b.** 65410

    **c.** 65410 and 65285 (in this order)

    **d.** None of these

**14.** [LO 12.6.4] The code for an incision for implantation of a cranial nerve neurostimulator electrode array and pulse generator is _____.

**a.** 64569

**b.** 64569 and 64570 (in this order)

**c.** 64568

**d.** 61885

**15.** [LO 12.6.4] Destruction by neurolytic agent, paravertebral facet joint nerve; sacral, single level, bilateral, is _____.

**a.** 64635, 64636

**b.** 64635-50

**c.** 64635 ×2

**d.** All of these

**16.** [LO 12.6.3] Neurolytic substance injection into the epidural region of the sacral level is coded as _____.

**a.** 62280

**b.** 62281

**c.** 62311

**d.** 62282

**17.** [LO 12.6.3] Hemilaminectomy with decompression of nerve roots, foraminotomy, and excision of herniated disc, L4–5, is coded as _____.

**a.** 63017

**b.** 63012

**c.** 63030

**d.** 63042

**18.** [LO 12.6.2] Puncture of shunt reservoir for aspiration with radiological supervision and interpretation is coded as _____.

**a.** 61070

**b.** 61070-26

**c.** 61070 and 75809

**d.** 61070 and 75800

**19.** [LO 12.6.2] Suboccipital craniectomy for mesencephalic tractotomy is coded as _____.

**a.** 61470

**b.** 61480

**c.** 61458 and 61480 (in this order)

**d.** None of these

## Applying Your Skills

Using your CPT manual, assign the appropriate code(s) to describe each procedure.

**1.** [LO 12.6.2] Initial bilateral subdural tap through fontanelle on an infant. _____

**2.** [LO 12.6.2] Craniotomy for drainage of intracranial abscess, infratentorial. _____

**3.** [LO 12.6.2] Exploration of orbit, transcranial approach, with removal of lesion. _____

**4.** [LO 12.6.3] Diagnostic percutaneous aspiration within paravertebral tissue. _____

**5.** [LO 12.6.3] Revision of tunneled epidural catheter for long-term medication via an external pump, with laminectomy. _____

**6.** [LO 12.6.4] Injection of anesthetic agent into the vagus nerve. _____

**7.** [LO 12.6.4] Application of transcutaneous neurostimulator. _____

**8.** [LO 12.6.4] Neuroplasty of the sciatic nerve via open incision. _____

**9.** [LO 12.6.5] Enucleation of eye with implant, muscles attached to implant. _____

**10.** [LO 12.6.5] Repair of laceration of conjunctiva by mobilization and rearrangement. _____

## Case Studies

Read each case study. Using your CPT manual, assign the appropriate code(s) to describe each case.

**1.** [LO 12.6.1] A patient presented for incision and drainage of an infected thyrolingual cyst. The cyst was incised and the infected fluid was drained. The wound was irrigated with normal saline, and drainage tubes were sutured in place. Code the incision and drainage procedure.

_____

**2.** [LO 12.6.1] A 41-year-old significantly overweight female was suffering from weight gain, and extreme physical lethargy prevented her from engaging in an active lifestyle. The patient was diagnosed with hypothyroidism. She subsequently underwent a total thyroidectomy. Code the procedure.

_____

**3.** [LO 12.6.2] A 32-year-old hospitalized trauma patient in the ICU was showing signs of an abnormal accumulation of cerebrospinal fluid. The patient had an established burr hole from a previous procedure. The physician performed a ventricular puncture through this same burr hole and placed a ventricular catheter. Fluid was withdrawn for study in order to establish a diagnosis. Code the ventricular puncture and placement of the ventricular catheter.

_____

**4.** [LO 12.6.2] The following morning, this same patient, still hospitalized in the ICU, was diagnosed with meningitis. Via ventricular puncture and the already implanted catheter, antibiotic medication was administered. Code the injection of medication for treatment via the ventricular catheter.

_____

**5.** [LO 12.6.2] A 61-year-old patient underwent cranial stereotactic radiosurgery for the therapeutic creation of two cranial lesions. One cranial lesion measured 3.4 cm at its greatest diameter and the second, 3.7 cm.

_____

**6.** [LO 12.6.3] A 27-year-old female was admitted for an outpatient percutaneous needle biopsy of the spinal cord. With the patient in the "spinal tap position," the surgeon administered a local anesthetic and placed the needle into the T1–T2 disc interspace. A tissue sample from the lesion was obtained and sent for pathological examination. Code the percutaneous needle biopsy.

_____

**7.** [LO 12.6.6] While operating a chainsaw and cutting a limb off a tree, a 31-year-old male fell off a ladder propped against the tree. As he fell, his right ear was severely cut and barely connected to his head. The patient was airlifted via trauma helicopter to the hospital. His ear was amputated by scalpel. Reconstruction procedure(s) would be done after healing at the site of the amputation. Code the amputation only.

_____

## Thinking It Through

Using your critical-thinking skills, answer the following questions.

**1.** [LO 12.6.5] Why would Medicare and or other payers want Level II modifiers used with CPT procedure codes, such as those describing procedures on the eye?

_____

_____

_____

_____

**2.** [LO 12.6.2]  In reading code descriptions, coders frequently have to research medical terms or anatomy. Is there a difference between excision of somatic nerves and excision of sympathetic nerves? Describe the nerve characteristics, and indicate what makes them similar and dissimilar. Refer to CPT codes 64774–64823.

_____

_____

_____

_____

**3.** [LO 12.6.5]  Lens removal procedures of the eye are intracapsular, such as CPT codes 66920–66930, or extracapsular, such as CPT code 66940. What is the difference between intracapsular and extracapsular procedures?

_____

_____

_____

_____

## Learning Outcomes

*After completing this chapter, students should be able to:*

**13.1** Differentiate between organ-oriented and disease-oriented panels and the individual codes used to report those tests.

**13.2** Explain how to report laboratory tests related to drugs and medicines.

**13.3** Identify codes to report laboratory tests.

**13.4** Select appropriate codes to describe pathology services.

## Introduction

Pathology and laboratory tests provide important information necessary for practitioners to diagnose and treat patients. Laboratory tests may be performed on specimens from many sources, including blood, urine, or small amounts of tissues or fluids from any anatomical location. Laboratory tests may be either qualitative or quantitative. Qualitative tests show whether a substance is present in the specimen or not. Their results may be thought of as +/−, true/false, or yes/no. On the other hand, quantitative tests reveal how much of a substance is present in the specimen. Their results are numerical. This allows comparisons over time of any changes in those results, which may be necessary to monitor the results of treatment and changes in the overall health of patients. CPT codes describing these tests are grouped into large sections.

Pathology procedures are divided into two types— anatomical and surgical. Anatomical pathology is the postmortem examination of a body and the various organs. It includes gross examination (visual examination and measurements only) and microscopic examinations in which tissues are prepared and examined at the cellular level. Surgical pathology involves the examination of tissues removed from a person as part of treatment to determine the type and severity of disease present in the sample. These tests may be done while a patient is still in surgery, if the surgical procedure depends on those results, or after surgery to provide additional information necessary to confirm the diagnosis or determine the course of follow-up treatment.

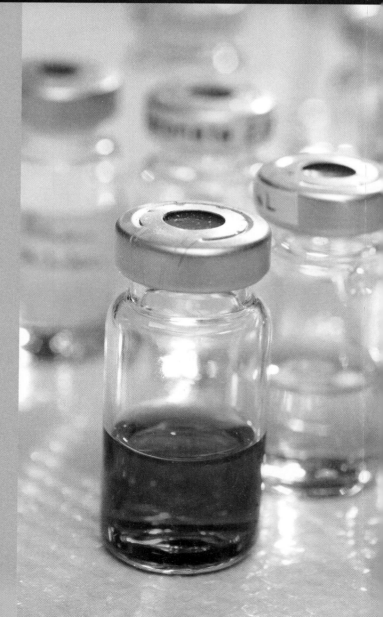

# Key Terms

Define each of the following key terms in the space provided.

**1.** [LO 13.4]  Anatomic pathology _____

_____

**2.** [LO 13.1]  Chemistry _____

_____

**3.** [LO 13.3]  Complete blood count (CBC) _____

_____

**4.** [LO 13.2]  Drug test _____

_____

**5.** [LO 13.2]  Evocative/suppression testing _____

_____

**6.** [LO 13.1]  Laboratory _____

_____

**7.** [LO 13.3]  Microscopy _____

_____

**8.** [LO 13.1]  Organ/disease panel _____

_____

**9.** [LO 13.3]  Partial thromboplastin time (PTT) _____

_____

**10.** [LO 13.3]  Prothrombin time (PT) _____

_____

**11.** [LO 13.2]  Qualitative _____

_____

**12.** [LO 13.2]  Quantitative _____

_____

**13.** [LO 13.3]  Red blood cell (RBC) _____

_____

**14.** [LO 13.3]  Specimen _____

_____

**15.** [LO 13.4]  Surgical pathology _____

_____

**16.** [LO 13.2]  Therapeutic level _____

_____

**17.** [LO 13.3]  Urinalysis (UA) _____

_____

**18.** [LO 13.3]  White blood cell (WBC) _____

_____

# Exam Review

Select the letter that best completes the statement or answers the question.

**1.** [LO 13.1]  Which of the following is *not* true regarding organ- and disease-oriented panels?
   **a.** They may be used to screen for disease.
   **b.** They were developed for coding purposes.
   **c.** They serve as clinical guidelines for appropriate tests.
   **d.** They may be used to diagnose disease.

**2.** [LO 13.1]  Organ- or disease-oriented panels may only be reported if _____ tests in the panel have been performed.
   **a.** Some
   **b.** Drug
   **c.** All
   **d.** Chemistry

**3.** [LO 13.1]  AST, ALT, and direct bilirubin are all included on which panel?
   **a.** Basic metabolic panel
   **b.** Hepatic function panel
   **c.** Comprehensive metabolic panel
   **d.** General health panel

**4.** [LO 13.2]  A urine drug test that indicates positive or negative for cocaine is an example of _____.
   **a.** A qualitative test
   **b.** A quantitative test
   **c.** A therapeutic drug assay
   **d.** A qualitative drug panel

**5.** [LO 13.2]  A result of "9685 mIU/ml" for a human chorionic gonadotropin (HCG) test would indicate which type of test?
   **a.** Qualitative urine pregnancy test
   **b.** Therapeutic HCG level assay
   **c.** Qualitative serum pregnancy test
   **d.** Quantitative serum pregnancy test

**6.** [LO 13.2]  Which of the following is not an example of an evocative/suppression test, for which a person is administered the first substance and tested for the second substance?
   **a.** Testosterone, FSH
   **b.** Phenobarbital, phenytoin
   **c.** Glucagon, insulin
   **d.** Dexamethasone, cortisol

**7.** [LO 13.3]  Which urinalysis could be done entirely by a laboratory instrument without human intervention (other than preparation of the sample)?
   **a.** Nonautomated, with microscopy
   **b.** Automated, with microscopy
   **c.** Automated, without microscopy
   **d.** Nonautomated, without microscopy

**8.** [LO 13.3]  Which of the following tests is measured in time units?
   **a.** WBCs
   **b.** RBCs
   **c.** Platelets
   **d.** PT

9. [LO 13.3]  Which of the following is not an example of a blood type?
   **a.** AB
   **b.** Rh
   **c.** A
   **d.** O

10. [LO 13.3]  Testing for which of the following would be an example of a microbiology test?
    **a.** Eosinophilia
    **b.** Hemosiderin
    **c.** Borrelia
    **d.** Trisomy

11. [LO 13.3]  Which of the following gives a quantitative measure of blood clotting time?
    **a.** PT
    **b.** Platelets
    **c.** WBCs
    **d.** Warfarin level

12. [LO 13.3]  Which of the following is not a service under the transfusion medicine codes?
    **a.** Thawing of fresh frozen plasma
    **b.** Leukocyte transfusion
    **c.** Plasma apheresis
    **d.** Blood typing

13. [LO 13.4]  Which is an example of a valid anatomic pathology service?
    **a.** Microscopic evaluation of brain biopsy
    **b.** Gross examination of gallbladder after cholecystectomy
    **c.** Chromosomal studies on a miscarried fetus
    **d.** Limited postmortem examination of the heart

14. [LO 13.4]  A Pap smear is an example of what type of study?
    **a.** Surgical pathology
    **b.** Cytogenetic
    **c.** Cytopathology
    **d.** Microbiology

15. [LO 13.4]  Which of the following does *not* provide any determination of a surgical pathology code?
    **a.** Gross or microscopic examination
    **b.** Organ or body part under examination
    **c.** The weight of the sample being examined
    **d.** Probability of disease or malignancy

16. [LO 13.1]  A patient has a comprehensive metabolic panel, TSH, and a CBC with differential. Report code(s) _____.
    **a.** 80053, 84443, and 85025
    **b.** 80047 and 85025
    **c.** 80055
    **d.** 80050

17. [LO 13.1]  A physician orders a basic metabolic panel with ionized calcium and total calcium. Report code(s) _____.
    **a.** 80048
    **b.** 80047 and 82310
    **c.** 80047 and 80048
    **d.** 82330 and 82310

18. [LO 13.1] The laboratory performs all the components of a basic metabolic panel with total calcium and reports the results with the note: "Potassium 6.7, probably invalid due to hemolysis of sample." Report code(s) _____.
   a. 80048-52
   b. 82310, 82374, 82435, 82565, 82947, 84295, and 84520
   c. 80048
   d. 84132

19. [LO 13.2] A patient has a test for amitriptyline only (a tricyclic antidepressant) with the result of "positive." Report code _____.
   a. 80101
   b. 80152
   c. 80100
   d. 80102

20. [LO 13.2] A patient with osteomyelitis has a vancomycin level measured before and after receiving an IV dose of the antibiotic to establish the "peak and trough" levels. Report code(s) _____.
   a. 80202 and 80102
   b. 80202 ×2
   c. 80202 and 80101
   d. 80202

21. [LO 13.2] An emergency department patient with abdominal pain has a positive serum pregnancy test followed by a serum HCG level as a baseline for future levels. Report code(s) _____.
   a. 81025 and 84702
   b. 84702
   c. 84703 and 84704
   d. 84703 and 84702

22. [LO 13.2] Dennis is worked up for insulinoma by receiving glucagon IV followed by both glucose and insulin levels at one hour, two hours, and four hours postinjection. Report code(s) _____.
   a. 80432
   b. 80422
   c. 82947 ×3 and 83525 ×3
   d. 80422 ×3

23. [LO 13.3] A rural family physician performs a dipstick urinalysis and microscopic examination to check for prostatitis. Report code(s) _____.
   a. 81000
   b. 81001
   c. 81000 and 81007
   d. 81099

24. [LO 13.3] Lois presents with mysterious and prolonged abdominal pains. Her physician has a qualitative serum arsenic test performed. Report code _____.
   a. 83015
   b. 83018
   c. 82175
   d. 82180

25. [LO 13.3] Bridget has unexplained bruising. Her physician orders a bleeding time. Report code _____.
   a. 85049
   b. 85002
   c. 85610
   d. 85175

26. [LO 13.4] A patient with biopsy-proved breast cancer has a mastectomy with regional lymph node excision. All tissue is sent for pathology. For the pathology service, report code(s) _____.

   **a.** 88307
   **b.** 88307 ×2
   **c.** 88307 and 88309
   **d.** 88309

27. [LO 13.4] Mr. Francis is shot in the chest and dies in the ER. A limited autopsy is performed on the chest to determine which specific organ injury was the cause of death. Report code _____.

   **a.** 88000
   **b.** 88306
   **c.** 88045
   **d.** 88020

28. [LO 13.3] Wallace presents with penile discharge and has a culture performed for chlamydia. Report code _____.

   **a.** 87270
   **b.** 87320
   **c.** 87110
   **d.** 86631

29. [LO 13.4] A kidney biopsy is obtained on a transplant patient to check for rejection. A hospital pathology lab prepares the specimen for examination and sends it to a specialty center for the actual pathological evaluation. For the hospital pathology services report code _____.

   **a.** 88305-TC
   **b.** 88305-26
   **c.** 88305
   **d.** 88305-52

30. [LO 13.4] During a gastric bypass surgery, Mrs. Ianello's liver is noted to have an unusual color. A pathologist is called into the OR for an intraoperative consultation during the actual surgery. She inspects the liver and advises this is a normal variation and not indicative of a problem. The gastric bypass procedure is completed without further attention to the liver. For the pathology service only report code _____.

   **a.** 88325
   **b.** 88331
   **c.** 88321
   **d.** 88329

## Applying Your Skills

Using your CPT manual, provide codes for the following pathology and laboratory services. Include any necessary modifiers.

1. [LO 13.1] Acute hepatitis panel. _____
2. [LO 13.1] Obstetric panel. _____
3. [LO 13.2] Growth hormone stimulation panel. _____
4. [LO 13.3] Serum cocaine level. _____
5. [LO 13.2] Serum gold assay. _____
6. [LO 13.2] Drugs of abuse screen, testing for five classes, chromatographic method, one stationary and one mobile phase for each. _____
7. [LO 13.2] Serum MDMA (ecstasy) level screening. _____
8. [LO 13.3] Microscopic examination (only) of urine. _____
9. [LO 13.3] Screening for arsenic, barium, beryllium, bismuth, antimony, and mercury. _____
10. [LO 13.3] Copper sulfate manual test to determine hemoglobin level. _____

**11.** [LO 13.3] Automated CBC with differential. _____

**12.** [LO 13.3] Quantitative test for IgE due to sequoia pollen exposure. _____

**13.** [LO 13.4] Surgical pathology on a hydrocele sac. _____

**14.** [LO 13.4] Diagnostic electron microscopy. _____

**15.** [LO 13.4] Test of sperm motility and count. _____

## Case Studies

Read each case study. Using your CPT manual, assign the appropriate code(s) to describe each case.

**1.** [LO 13.1]  Mr. McPeak presents to the emergency department with jaundice and has a hepatic function panel, a comprehensive metabolic panel, and an acute hepatitis panel performed.

_____

**2.** [LO 13.2]  A physician orders a four-class drug panel on a patient, and the panel is positive for benzodiazepines. This is followed by separate confirmatory tests for alprazolam, lorazepam, and diazepam.

_____

**3.** [LO 13.2]  Nine-year-old Mark is admitted to the hospital to determine the cause of his unusually small stature. His physician orders a growth hormone stimulation panel, and Mark is given IV doses of arginine and L-dopa, and has six separate tests for human growth hormone.

_____

**4.** [LO 13.2]  A patient on multiple medications for seizure disorder has blood drawn for routine monitoring of levels of phenobarbital and valproic acid.

_____

**5.** [LO 13.3]  An infant with fever and vomiting has an automated CBC with differential, basic metabolic panel (calcium, ionized), and automated urinalysis with microscopy. This shows an infection, and therefore a urine culture with bacterial identification is also performed.

_____

**6.** [LO 13.3]  Francesco is seen by an otolaryngologist for prolonged sinusitis a few months after his house had been severely flooded. The physician performs an *Aspergillus* antibody test, which is positive, followed by a fungal culture of the patient's nose to confirm the infection.

_____

**7.** [LO 13.3]  Richard develops a cough and fever six months after moving to Arizona. His family doctor performs a skin test for valley fever (coccidioidomycosis) and orders an automated CBC to check his white blood cell count and differential.

_____

**8.** [LO 13.4]  Mrs. Barnes has three consecutive miscarriages. Her obstetrician suspects a chromosomal abnormality causing a congenital problem. The doctor orders examination of the fetal tissue limited to chromosome analysis with karyotype.

_____

**9.** [LO 13.4]  A patient with primary hyperparathyroidism has surgical excision of a suspected parathyroid adenoma. During surgery a single frozen section pathology study is performed, confirming the adenoma is benign. Permanent surgical pathology is also performed and requires a decalcification procedure to obtain a valid tissue sample for microscopic study. Report only the pathology code(s).

_____

**10.** [LO 13.4]  A semen sample is analyzed for motility and Huhner test. After the sample is assessed as being adequate, it is then used for microtechnique-assisted fertilization of 20 oocytes, which are then held for extended culture for six days.

_____

# Thinking It Through

Using your critical-thinking skills, answer the questions below.

**1.** [LO 13.1] Describe the reason for developing the organ and disease-oriented panels and their intended usage.

_____

_____

_____

_____

**2.** [LO 13.2] Distinguish between a qualitative and a quantitative lab test, and give one example.

_____

_____

_____

_____

**3.** [LO 13.3] In identifying infections in their patients, clinicians may use microbiology tests or antibody tests. Define the code ranges for each of these categories, and describe some of the differences between the tests.

_____

_____

_____

_____

**4.** [LO 13.4] What are the levels and code ranges for surgical pathology (gross and microscopy), and why is it important for the coder to understand the exact source and composition of the sample?

_____

_____

_____

_____

**5.** [LO 13.2] Describe two unique qualities of the evocative and suppression testing code category.

_____

_____

_____

_____

## Learning Outcomes

*After completing this chapter, students should be able to:*

**14.1** Explain the structure of the Medicine section and its general guidelines.

**14.2** Select codes to report the administration of immune globulins and vaccines.

**14.3** Identify codes to report psychiatry, dialysis, gastroenterology, ophthalmology, and otorhinolaryngological services.

**14.4** Select codes to report cardiovascular, immunological, and neurological procedures.

**14.5** Identify codes to report injections, infusions, therapeutic procedures, rehabilitation, moderate sedation, home health services, and medication therapeutic management.

## Introduction

The Medicine section (90000 series) is a collection of many types of codes that do not fit neatly into other sections of the CPT manual. In this section, there are over 30 separate subsections and more than 100 sub-subsections of codes. A few of the larger subsections include vaccines, psychiatric services, dialysis, ophthalmology, cardiovascular services, diagnostic and therapeutic coronary catheterization, and fluid and medication administration. Adjacent code subsections may not be related to one another either anatomically or by types of services.

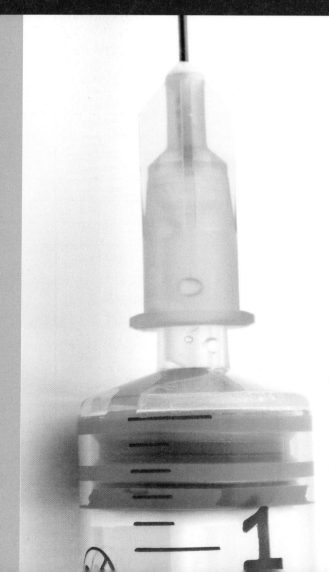

# Key Terms

Define each of the following key terms in the space provided.

**1.** [LO 14.2]  Administration _____

_____

**2.** [LO 14.3]  Bronchodilator _____

_____

**3.** [LO 14.3]  Aphakia _____

_____

**4.** [LO 14.4]  Cardiography _____

_____

**5.** [LO 14.4]  Cardiac catheterization _____

_____

**6.** [LO 14.4]  Congenital _____

_____

**7.** [LO 14.4]  Coronary artery stent _____

_____

**8.** [LO 14.4]  Electroencephalogram _____

_____

**9.** [LO 14.2]  Human papilloma virus (HPV) _____

_____

**10.** [LO 14.2]  Immune globulin _____

_____

**11.** [LO 14.2]  Measles, mumps, and rubella (MMR) _____

_____

**12.** [LO 14.5]  Moderate sedation _____

_____

**13.** [LO 14.3]  Refractive state _____

_____

**14.** [LO 14.2]  Vaccine _____

_____

# Exam Review

Select the letter that best completes the statement or answers the question.

**1.** [LO 14.5]  Which increment of face-to-face contact time is reported when performing acupuncture?

   **a.** 10 minutes
   **b.** 15 minutes
   **c.** 20 minutes
   **d.** 30 minutes

**2.** [LO 14.2]  Immune globulin codes (90281–90399) do not use modifier _____.

   **a.** 26                  **c.** 51
   **b.** 47                  **d.** 22

3. [LO 14.1] Some procedures and services classified in the Medicine section are considered an integral component of a complete procedure or service, but may sometimes be performed as the only procedure. These are identified by the description _____.
   a. Add-on codes
   b. Special report
   c. Home health procedures and services
   d. Separate procedure

4. [LO 14.3] Code 90968 is reported each day when less than a full month of ESRD services is provided to a patient between _____ years.
   a. 2 and 11
   b. 11 and 16
   c. 0 and 2
   d. 5 and 10

5. [LO 14.1] When no surgical incision or excision is required to perform a procedure, it is considered _____.
   a. Minimally invasive
   b. Noninvasive
   c. An add-on code
   d. A separate procedure

6. [LO 14.1] The Medicine section includes most of the 90000 series of CPT codes. The exception is the series of codes that describe _____ services.
   a. Anesthesia
   b. E/M
   c. Pathology and laboratory
   d. Radiology

7. [LO 14.1] Procedures designated by add-on codes, identified by a plus (+) sign, can only be reported with a(n) _____.
   a. Parent code
   b. Separate procedure code
   c. HCPCS services
   d. Unlisted service or procedure

8. [LO 14.3] How often are CPT codes describing ESRD services reported?
   a. Weekly
   b. Monthly
   c. Annually
   d. Quarterly

9. [LO 14.2] The two codes reported for each vaccine given are:
   a. Vaccine and administration
   b. Vaccine and E/M service
   c. Vaccine and materials supplied by the physician
   d. Vaccine and the allergy extract

10. [LO 14.5] CPT codes that provide additional information regarding anesthesia services and are reported in addition to specific anesthesia services codes are _____.
    a. 99100, 99116, 99135, and 99140          c. 99100, 99116, 00100, and 01999
    b. 00100–01999                             d. None of these

11. [LO 14.3] CPT codes describing end-stage renal disease–related services for dialysis provided for less than a full month are differentiated by a patient's _____.
    a. Diagnosis          c. Symptoms
    b. Age                d. Treatment

12. [LO 14.3] Which of the following is not an example of an ophthalmology service covered under codes 92015–92287?
    a. Gonioscopy
    b. Topography
    c. Tomography
    d. Tonometry

13. [LO 14.3] Specific electrocardiographic monitoring codes exist for each of these time intervals except _____.
    a. 1 day
    b. 90 days
    c. 30 days
    d. 10 days

14. [LO 14.5] Which of the following services does *not* have an associated injection/infusion code family?
    a. Chemotherapy
    b. Hydration
    c. Therapeutic
    d. Anesthetic

15. [LO 14.5] For coding purposes, whole body photography monitoring for skin cancer would be an example of which category of special service.
    a. Photography
    b. Radiology
    c. Dermatology
    d. Part of E/M coding and not coded separately

16. [LO 14.2] An adult patient who has cut his hand receives an intramuscular tetanus toxoid booster. This is reported with code(s) _____.
    a. 90703
    b. 90471
    c. 90718 and 90471
    d. 90703 and 90471

17. [LO 14.3] A psychiatrist provides outpatient interactive psychotherapy to a new 10-year-old patient for 50 minutes and diagnoses ADHD. After reviewing the patient's records and laboratory results, she prescribes a stimulant medication. Report code(s) _____.
    a. 90812
    b. 90813
    c. 90812 and 90813
    d. 90807

18. [LO 14.3] A 16-year-old patient with complete renal failure receives 30 days of maintenance care services from her nephrologist, including one visit each week to evaluate dialysis services. What is the code?
    a. 90969
    b. 90965
    c. 90957
    d. 90959

19. [LO 14.3] Mr. Zellman, a 52 year-old patient, goes to a new ophthalmologist for a basic eye checkup including single-measurement tonometry for glaucoma screening. This is reported with code _____ from the Ophthalmology section.
    a. 92002
    b. 92004
    c. 92140
    d. 92100

**20.** [LO 14.4] A 1-month-old infant born with a known patent foramen ovale (PFO) has a limited follow-up transthoracic echocardiogram that shows the PFO has closed. Report code _____.
   **a.** 93303
   **b.** 93304
   **c.** 93312
   **d.** 93321

**21.** [LO 14.5] An obese patient with snoring undergoes a comprehensive polysomnography study with sleep staging. After four hours it is clear the patient has obstructive sleep apnea so the technologist initiates CPAP therapy. What code should be used to report the service?
   **a.** 95807
   **b.** 95808
   **c.** 95810
   **d.** 95811

**22.** [LO 14.5] Jamal receives an IV infusion of ceftriaxone (an antibiotic) over the course of two hours. What are the codes?
   **a.** 96365 and 96367
   **b.** 96365 and 96366
   **c.** 96365 and 96368
   **d.** 96365 and 96365

**23.** [LO 14.5] Andy presents with elbow tendonitis and receives an initial physical therapy evaluation and 30 minutes of direct, supervised therapeutic ultrasound over the affected tendon. Which code(s) should be used to report?
   **a.** 97001, 97035 ×2
   **b.** 97001 and 97035
   **c.** 97001
   **d.** 97002, 97035 ×2

**24.** [LO 14.5] An emergency room physician provides moderate sedation services on a 4-year-old child for 45 minutes while a plastic surgeon repairs a cat bite laceration to the child's cheek and mouth. List the codes for *only* the ER physician's services.
   **a.** 99143 and 99144
   **b.** 99143 and 99145
   **c.** 99148 and 99150
   **d.** 99149 and 99150

**25.** [LO 14.2] Mrs. Rachlin, a 69-year-old COPD patient, receives a Pneumovax (pneumococcal vaccine, 7-valent) shot at an annual checkup to reduce the risk of pneumonia. Which code(s) should be used to report the service(s)?
   **a.** 90669
   **b.** 90669 and 90471
   **c.** 90670
   **d.** 90670 and 90471

**26.** [LO 14.3] Hector, an alcoholic, attends a psychotherapy session with his family and close friends. What is the code?
   **a.** 90853
   **b.** 90846
   **c.** 90857
   **d.** 90847

**27.** [LO 14.3] As part of a "brain-death evaluation" on a comatose patient, Dr. Cooper performs a thorough caloric vestibular testing. This requires irrigating first cold and then warm water individually into each ear and observing the resulting eye movement. Code(s) _____ should be used to report this service.
   **a.** 92533
   **b.** 92533 × 4
   **c.** 92531 and 92533
   **d.** 92542

**28.** [LO 14.3] Three weeks after her cataract surgery to remove both of the diseased lenses, Vanessa visits her ophthalmologist for a corneal contact lens prescription for both eyes. Code(s) _____ should be used to report the service.

   **a.** 92310
   **b.** 92311 ×2
   **c.** 92312
   **d.** 92316

**29.** [LO 14.4] A rural physician personally performs an EKG on a patient presenting with chest pain. Using his antiquated machine, the physician interprets the three-lead EKG as showing a myocardial infarction. He generates a written report and summons an ambulance. Report code _____.

   **a.** 93040
   **b.** 93041
   **c.** 93000
   **d.** 93010

**30.** [LO 14.4] A patient experiencing a sudden worsening of his congestive heart failure is taken to the cardiac catheterization lab and undergoes diagnostic right heart catheterization and retrograde left heart catheterization to precisely measure his heart function. Report code(s) _____.

   **a.** 93451
   **b.** 93451 and 93452
   **c.** 93542
   **d.** 93453

## Applying Your Skills

Using your CPT manual, assign the appropriate code(s) for each medicine service. Include any necessary modifiers.

   **1.** [LO 14.2] Oral poliovirus administration. _____

   **2.** [LO 14.3] Fifty-minute inpatient psychotherapy session with a medical evaluation. _____

   **3.** [LO 14.3] Complete ophthalmology evaluation with patient under general anesthesia. _____

   **4.** [LO 14.4] Percutaneous transcatheter placement of a single intracoronary stent on a single coronary vessel. _____

   **5.** [LO 14.5] Continuous ambulatory subcutaneous interstitial glucose monitoring for 84 hours.
   _____

   **6.** [LO 14.5] Intralesional chemotherapy administration for nine distinct lesions on a patient. _____

   **7.** [LO 14.5] Occupational therapist's reevaluation of a patient. _____

   **8.** [LO 14.5] Home visit to evaluate a newborn. _____

   **9.** [LO 14.2] Hepatitis B IM vaccination for dialysis patient. _____

   **10.** [LO 14.5] Three hours of IV hydration while in the hospital. _____

   **11.** [LO 14.3] Peritoneal dialysis, with physician evaluation before, during, and after the procedure. _____

   **12.** [LO 14.3] Treatment for an auditory processing disorder. _____

   **13.** [LO 14.4] Overseeing management of a mechanical ventilator on a hospital patient for four days.
   _____

   **14.** [LO 14.4] Needle electromyography for both arms and legs. _____

   **15.** [LO 14.5] Third-degree burns over a 29 sq cm surface area of a patient's hand, treated by selective debridement and whirlpool of the burned area. _____

# Case Studies

Read each case study. Using your CPT manual, assign the appropriate code(s) to describe each case.

**1.** [LO 14.2] While on vacation in Honduras and after being bitten on the leg by a stray dog, 23-year-old Jaden presents to the emergency department. As prophylaxis against rabies the physician administers an intramuscular injection of rabies immune globulin (RIg) in the wound, an initial dose of rabies vaccine intramuscular in the right deltoid, plus a tetanus-diphtheria (Td) booster immunization in the left deltoid. List the codes for all services provided.

_____

**2.** [LO 14.3] A 21-year-old with a rare autoimmune disorder develops ESRD and is put on a kidney transplant list. She receives outpatient care (twice weekly visits from a nephrologist for 33 days) and is then hospitalized and immediately receives a kidney transplant. List report codes for the nephrologist's outpatient management services.

_____

**3.** [LO 14.3] Peter presents with deteriorating hearing and undergoes pure-tone audiometry of bone and air conduction plus speech audiometry with speech recognition measurement. To further refine the diagnosis, he has electrocochleography and a Stenger speech test. What are the codes for the services provided?

_____

**4.** [LO 14.4] Mrs. Kelsey is diagnosed in the ER with an acute myocardial infarction and is rushed to the cardiac catheterization lab. She undergoes left heart catheterization with ventriculography and angiography of the coronary arteries. The left anterior descending (LAD) and circumflex arteries are blocked. Percutaneous angioplasty is performed on these two vessels with deployment of two stents. What are the codes?

_____

**5.** [LO 14.4] An Iraq war veteran returns to the United States with a peculiar constellation of pulmonary symptoms, including wheezing, tightness, and coughing up gray mucus. He undergoes complex pulmonary stress testing followed by bronchospasm provocation testing with dust, mold, and cold air. Then he's tested for bronchodilation responsiveness with spirometry before and after albuterol administration. What are the codes?

_____

**6.** [LO 14.5] A patient with breast cancer receives IV chemotherapy for three hours, plus a single IV injection of diphenhydramine to reduce itching from the chemotherapy and a single IV injection of promethazine to help with nausea. What are the codes?

_____

**7.** [LO 14.5] Mr. Tami is seven days postop after a complex tendon reconstruction, and visits his physical therapist. He has 30 minutes of unattended whirlpool therapy to clean the surgical wound of scab and debris followed by 30 minutes of attended manual electrostimulation to strengthen the muscle and 30 minutes of therapeutic exercises to promote flexibility. What code(s) should be used to report these services?

_____

**8.** [LO 14.5] A quadriplegic patient, who has recently been discharged from a rehabilitation hospital, requires daily visits from a home care nurse. Each day the nurse performs evaluation on the patient's mechanical ventilator, provides a nebulized bronchodilator treatment, bathes the patient (personal care), drains and changes the urinary catheter drainage bag, and performs an infusion of antibiotic over three hours. What code(s) should be used to report one day of these services?

_____

**9.** [LO 14.2] A 2-year-old patient sees her pediatrician for routine immunizations and receives DTaP, MMR, and OPV. Assign codes for these immunizations.

_____

**10.** [LO 14.4] Mr. Gardner has a noninvasive electrophysiologic evaluation and programming of his dual-chamber pacing cardioverter-defibrillator, including defibrillation threshold evaluation, induction of arrhythmia, evaluation of sensing and pacing for arrhythmia termination, and reprogramming of sensing parameters. How would the service be reported?

_____

# Thinking It Through

Using your critical-thinking skills, answer the questions below.

**1.** [LO 14.2]  Describe the coding requirements for immunizations, particularly multiple administrations.

_____

_____

_____

_____

**2.** [LO 14.3]  What are four determinations a coder must make when coding for psychotherapy services?

_____

_____

_____

**3.** [LO 14.4]  List some procedures that may be performed with percutaneous coronary artery stent procedures. Designate whether they are reported in addition to the stent procedure.

_____

_____

_____

_____

**4.** [LO 14.5]  What details about injections and infusions of therapeutic agents must a coder know to accurately determine the codes to report?

_____

_____

_____

_____

**5.** [LO 14.5]  What information must a coder determine about physical medicine and rehabilitation services to report the correct codes?

_____

_____

_____

_____

## Learning Outcomes

*After completing this chapter, students should be able to:*

**15.1** Explain HCPCS codes.

**15.2** Identify services described by A-, B-, C-, and E-codes.

**15.3** Select codes to report services described by G-, H-, J-, K-, L-, and M-codes.

**15.4** Determine codes to report services described by P-, Q-, R-, S-, T-, and V-codes.

**15.5** Use HCPCS modifiers.

## Introduction

CPT codes identify services provided by physicians and other healthcare professionals. The Centers for Medicare and Medicaid Services (CMS) maintains a separate coding system, known as the Healthcare Common Procedure Coding System (HCPCS), to describe many services provided to patients other than professional medical services. HCPCS codes describe a wide variety of services, including medical supplies, transportation, durable medical equipment, orthotics and prosthetics, certain types of drugs, and nonprofessional services. Many providers, including professionals, use HCPCS codes to report some services. Because of the widespread use of HCPCS codes, coders must be familiar with HCPCS codes and how to use them correctly to report services in any healthcare setting.

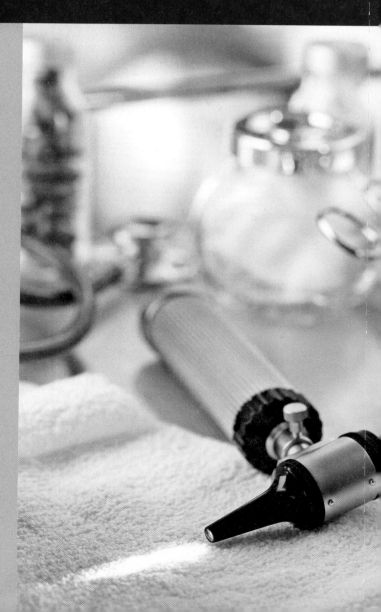

# Key Terms

Fill in the blanks with the correct key term.

**1.** _____ A device that generally replaces a missing body part.

**2.** _____ Current Procedural Terminology (CPT) codes that primarily describe services provided by physicians and other healthcare professionals.

**3.** _____ A particular amount of a described service included in a HCPCS code descriptor.

**4.** _____ The level of medical care given to patients with life-threatening illnesses or injuries until the patient reaches a hospital.

**5.** _____ Codes maintained and copyrighted by the American Dental Association that describe all dental services.

**6.** _____ Table in the HCPCS manual used to identify specific codes that describe medications provided to patients in physician offices or medical facilities.

**7.** _____ A device that supports an impaired body part.

**8.** _____ Transportation used to bring a critically ill patient to a hospital.

**9.** _____ Codes that report services, supplies, and equipment covered by Medicare and other insurers but that are not identified by CPT codes.

**10.** _____ Transportation used to move a patient who is not in immediate, critical need of medical care.

**11.** _____ Measures created for physicians in reporting their performance of certain services or the reason the service was not performed.

**12.** _____ A higher level of medical care that supports circulation and breathing while the patient is being transported.

**13.** _____ Items provided to patients as part of their treatments, generally used once and then disposed of.

**14.** _____ The provision of nutrients to prevent or treat malnutrition.

**15.** _____ Reusable medical equipment bought or rented for use in the home.

# Exam Review

Select the letter that best completes the statement or answers the question.

**1.** [LO 15.1] How many characters are commonly used to code for HCPCS Level II?
   **a.** Three
   **b.** Four
   **c.** Five
   **d.** Six

**2.** [LO 15.1] What is the proper procedure to follow when both CPT-4 and HCPCS codes have similar descriptors?
   **a.** Always use CPT-4 code.
   **b.** Always use HCPCS code.
   **c.** Use code which has most specific descriptor to procedure or item.
   **d.** Always use both.

**3.** [LO 15.1] Why is it important to pay attention to units when coding HCPCS?
   **a.** It is not important. HCPCS codes are general in nature.
   **b.** Coder must code to highest available unit or quantity without using units.
   **c.** Many HCPCS codes are limited to specific quantities for each description and must include units along with code.
   **d.** HCPCS codes do not utilize units.

**4.** [LO 15.3] When billing for Medicare, HCPCS _____ take precedence over CPT codes.
  **a.** A-codes
  **b.** C-codes
  **c.** G-codes
  **d.** V-codes

**5.** [LO 15.3] Which type of drug administration is covered under J-codes?
  **a.** Oral, parenteral, and topical
  **b.** Injection, infusion, and inhalation
  **c.** Transdermal, liquid, and injection
  **d.** All of these

**6.** [LO 15.4] When are R-codes utilized?
  **a.** They are stand-alone radiology codes for HCPCS.
  **b.** They take the place of CPT codes when coding for radiology services.
  **c.** They describe the transportation and setup of radiology equipment and are reported in conjunction with CPT or HCPCS codes that describe the radiology services.
  **d.** They are used in conjunction with E/M codes for radiological services.

**7.** [LO 15.4] It is appropriate to use a T-code _____.
  **a.** To identify anatomic locations
  **b.** To identify transportation
  **c.** To report tests performed by hospitals
  **d.** To report nursing and home health-related services to Medicaid agencies

**8.** [LO 15.5] Which anatomical modifiers indicate coronary arteries?
  **a.** E1–E4
  **b.** RC, LC, and LD
  **c.** FA and F1–F9
  **d.** None of these

**9.** [LO 15.2] How many sections (letters) are assigned to HCPCS Level II?
  **a.** 17                          **c.** 20
  **b.** 12                          **d.** 15

**10.** [LO 15.2] HCPCS _____ are generally used for items provided in an outpatient hospital setting.
  **a.** V-codes
  **b.** G-codes
  **c.** F-codes
  **d.** C-codes

**11.** [LO 15.3] Why must the coder be careful when assigning L-codes?
  **a.** Descriptors may be very similar to one another.
  **b.** Descriptors are similar to M-codes.
  **c.** You do not need to be careful; all descriptions are specific.
  **d.** Multiple codes may be needed to correctly identify the service.

**12.** [LO 15.3] When are L-codes assigned?
  **a.** For coding of pathology and laboratory services
  **b.** For coding of orthotic and prosthetic devices
  **c.** For in-home or caregiving services
  **d.** For miscellaneous rarely used services

**13.** [LO 15.2] Which code is used to report provision of wheelchair accessory, bearings only? This code must be used for each bearing.
  **a.** E2204                       **c.** E2206
  **b.** E2205                       **d.** E2210

14. [LO 15.3] Injection of five units of insulin is reported with code _____.
    a. J1815
    b. J1817
    c. J1825
    d. J1835

15. [LO 15.3] Oral administration of 2 mg melphalan is reported with code _____.
    a. J8520
    b. J8600
    c. J8610
    d. J8530

16. [LO 15.3] What is the code for a custom-fabricated cranial orthotic device with an adjustable range of motion joint, congenital torticollis type with soft interface material?
    a. L0113
    b. L0120
    c. L0112
    d. L0130

17. [LO 15.3] What is the code for a nonadjustable flexible cervical orthotic device (soft foam cervical collar)?
    a. L0113
    b. L0120
    c. L0112
    d. L0130

18. [LO 15.3] Immediate postsurgical fitting of a below-knee rigid dressing with one dressing change is reported with code _____.
    a. L5460
    b. L5410
    c. L5420
    d. L5400

19. [LO 15.2] What is the code for the second cast/dressing change of an immediate postsurgical fitting of a below-knee dressing?
    a. L5460
    b. L5410
    c. L5420
    d. L5400

20. [LO 15.4] A PAP smear screening test and evaluation, three slides, interpreted by a physician is reported with code _____.
    a. P2029
    b. P2038
    c. P3000
    d. P3001

21. [LO 15.4] Code _____ would be used to report a single vision lens, plano sphere with 0.12–2.00 cylinder per lens.
    a. V2102
    b. V2105
    c. V2103
    d. V2107

22. [LO 15.4] What is the code for a contact lens (gas permeable, spherical, per lens)?
    a. V2510
    b. V2511
    c. V2512
    d. V2513

**23.** [LO 15.2] The code for a nasal cannula is _____.

   **a.** A4616

   **b.** A4619

   **c.** A4615

   **d.** A4624

**24.** [LO 15.2] A hydrogel dressing, more than 48 sq in., without adhesive border, would be coded as _____.

   **a.** A6246

   **b.** A6247

   **c.** A6244

   **d.** A6245

**25.** [LO 15.2] Parenteral nutrition solution, 7.5 percent amino acid; 500 ml = 1U home mix, would be coded as _____.

   **a.** B4180

   **b.** B4178

   **c.** B4177

   **d.** B4176

## Applying Your Skills

Using your HCPCS manual, assign the appropriate code(s) for each service.

**1.** Minibus, nonemergency transportation. _____

**2.** Wound filler, hydrogel dressing. _____

**3.** Transportation, x-ray (portable). _____

**4.** Adrenalin. _____

**5.** Hot water bottle. _____

**6.** Hydraulic patient lift. _____

**7.** Negative pressure wound therapy pump. _____

**8.** WHO, wrist extension. _____

**9.** Peroneal straps, pair. _____

**10.** UV lens. _____

**11.** Bacterial sensitivity study. _____

**12.** Chair for bathtub. _____

**13.** Electrocardiographic monitoring, with physician supervision. _____

**14.** Therapy for osteoporosis. _____

**15.** Peripherally inserted central venous catheter (PICC) line insertion. _____

## Case Studies

Read each case study. Using your HCPCS manual, assign the appropriate code(s) to describe each case.

**1.** [LO 15.3] Sally, age 64, is suffering from enuresis and incontinence. Her physician recommends incontinence briefs, and prescribes two to start. Code the service.

_____

   

**2.** [LO 15.3]  Mr. Michaels was seen in the ER for severe back pain and given an injection of 5 mg hydromorphone. Code the service.

_____

**3.** [LO 15.3]  A physician provides Melissa, age 23, a levalbuterol 0.5 mg inhaler.

_____

**4.** [LO 15.3]  Robert Thomas, a paraplegic is traveling out of state and requires the use of a portable wheelchair. He needs it to be light but able to support his weight of 360 lb. Code the provision of Robert's wheelchair.

_____

**5.** [LO 15.3]  Mr. Baker suffers a C3 partial fracture requiring the administration of a cervical HALO with jacket vest. Code the service.

_____

**6.** [LO 15.3]  Jewel Sullivan was diagnosed with a condition causing her left leg to be 3.5 cm shorter than her right leg. This requires application of a 1 inch heel sole lift.

_____

**7.** [LO 15.3]  Mrs. Covington is S/P radical bilateral mastectomy and visits a DME supplier for the fitting of mastectomy bra with integrated breast prostheses. What code(s) are used to report?

_____

**8.** [LO 15.3]  Letitia visits a urologist complaining of dysuria, hematuria, fever, and flank pain. Her doctor orders bacterial culture of urine, quantitative. Which code(s) should be used to report the service?

_____

**9.** [LO 15.3]  An 88-year-old woman visits her ophthalmologist for a vision exam. She is prescribed a spherocylinder, single vision, 3.00d sphere 0.14 cylinder lens for her left eye and a spherocylinder, single vision, 5.28 cylinder lens for her right eye. Code the services.

_____

**10.** [LO 15.3]  Eddie, 4 years old, visits an audiologist to have a hearing screening.

_____

## Thinking It Through

Using your critical-thinking skills, answer the following questions.

**1.** [LO 15.1]  The Centers for Medicare and Medicaid Services maintains a separate coding system known as the Healthcare Common Procedure Coding System (HCPCS). Why is this system different from other coding systems?

_____

_____

_____

_____

**2.** [LO 15.2]  When coding for medications given by a physician in his office, you look at the index and the Table of Drugs in the HCPCS book. You locate the medication listed in the C-code section of the HCPCS book. Is it appropriate to report the C-code for the physician-administered medication? Why or why not?

_____

_____

_____

_____

**3.** [LO 15.2, LO 15.4] When reporting supplies provided to a Medicaid patient, you notice that there is a code that is similar in the A-code series and an exact match in the T-code section. Which code would be reported? Justify your choice.

_____

_____

_____

_____

**4.** [LO 15.1] When reporting services, you find that there is a CPT and a HCPCS code report the same service. Which code would be correct to report the service and why?

_____

_____

_____

_____

**5.** [LO 15.1] Why is it important to compare the number and type of units in HCPCS code descriptors to the services provided to patients?

_____

_____

_____

_____

_____

# PUTTING IT ALL TOGETHER

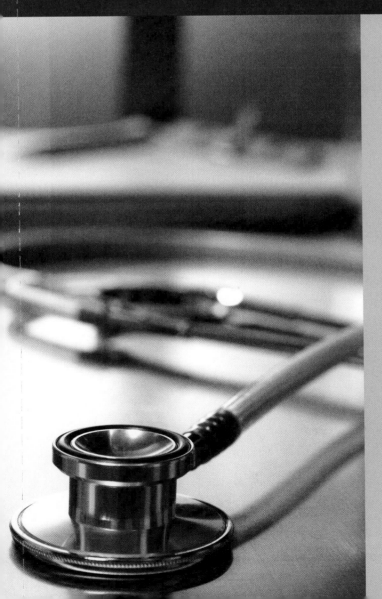

## Introduction

This chapter is the culmination of the material presented in the previous chapters of the book. At this point in your training, you should be able to select diagnosis, CPT, and HCPCS codes, as well as the appropriate modifiers, to describe services provided and the reasons they were necessary. Now it's time to put it all together and prepare for real-life coding by reviewing theory and assigning codes from all these sources. Because the questions in this chapter may refer to material from any chapter, and the answers might be found in any section of the manuals, prepare for these exercises by having your coding resources (manuals and reference materials) available.

# Key Terms

The following terms and word parts often appear in medical documentation. Define each of the following key terms in the space provided.

**1.** [LO 16.1]  Cholecystectomy _____

_____

**2.** [LO 16.1]  DM _____

_____

**3.** [LO 16.1]  CVA _____

_____

**4.** [LO 16.1]  ASHD _____

_____

**5.** [LO 16.1]  Dysphagia _____

_____

**6.** [LO 16.1]  Neoplasm _____

_____

**7.** [LO 16.1]  Chief complaint _____

_____

**8.** [LO 16.1]  General anesthesia _____

_____

**9.** [LO 16.1]  Base unit _____

_____

**10.** [LO 16.1]  Physical status modifier _____

_____

**11.** [LO 16.1]  PFSH _____

_____

**12.** [LO 16.1]  GERD _____

_____

**13.** [LO 16.1]  I&D _____

_____

**14.** [LO 16.1]  NKDA _____

_____

**15.** [LO 16.1]  ABG _____

_____

# Exam Review

Select the letter that best completes the statement or answers the question.

**1.** [LO 16.1]  Which of the following should be considered when coding from a case scenario or the patient's medical record?

    **a.** The patient's chief complaint or reason for the visit

    **b.** The place where services are rendered

    **c.** The coder's interpretation of laboratory or pathology reports

    **d.** Both (*a*) and (*b*)

2. [LO 16.1] Which of the following supports reporting a particular procedure code?
   **a.** A diagnosis code linked with the appropriate procedure code to support the reason the procedure was performed
   **b.** Medical record documentation that is thorough enough to substantiate that the particular procedure identified by the CPT code was the procedure performed by the provider
   **c.** Level III codes
   **d.** Both (*a*) and (*b*)

3. [LO 16.1] Which of the following determines the codes used to report a service?
   **a.** Place of service (POS)
   **b.** Patient's history
   **c.** Procedure performed
   **d.** All of the above

4. [LO 16.1] A coder uses _____ to specify that the procedure reported has been altered by some specific circumstance but the definition of the code has not changed.
   **a.** Modifiers
   **b.** CPT codes
   **c.** Diagnostic codes
   **d.** HCPCS codes

5. [LO 16.1] Which of the following must be reported when injections are administered to a patient?
   **a.** The physician who administered the injections or oversaw the procedure
   **b.** The nurse who administered the injections
   **c.** The number of injections provided
   **d.** Both (*a*) and (*c*)

6. [LO 16.1] Which medical records should be reviewed to accurately report services?
   **a.** Face sheet or emergency record
   **b.** Discharge summary
   **c.** History and physical
   **d.** All of the above

7. [LO 16.1] Which of the following must be considered when coding from a patient's medical record?
   **a.** Whether radiological supervision or interpretation was involved
   **b.** Whether add-on codes are required
   **c.** Whether the problem was an acute versus a chronic condition
   **d.** All of the above

8. [LO 16.1] Which of the following best determines the level of code to assign for evaluation and management of the patient?
   **a.** The complexity of medical decision making
   **b.** The level of examination performed
   **c.** The time spent with the patient
   **d.** Both (*a*) and (*b*)

9. [LO 16.1] When reading a case scenario and/or medical record documentation with many different diagnoses, which codes should the coder report?
   **a.** Report the codes that are treated during the encounter
   **b.** Report the codes that have an impact on the current encounter
   **c.** Report all codes, including those that have been previously treated and are no longer present
   **d.** Both (*a*) and (*b*)

10. [LO 16.1] The codes describing emergency helicopter transportation are found in the _____?
    **a.** HCPCS manual
    **b.** ICD coding manual
    **c.** CPT coding manual
    **d.** List of modifiers

11. [LO 16.1] Coders can find evaluation and management codes describing services provided in an emergency room in the _____?
    a. ICD coding manual
    b. CPT coding manual
    c. HCPCS coding manual
    d. Medical dictionary

12. [LO 16.1] When reading a case scenario and/or a patient's medical record, you can best code for procedures by doing which of the following?
    a. Identifying the main procedure term in the alphabetical index of the CPT coding manual and then reviewing the codes in the tabular list
    b. Identifying the main procedure in the tabular list and then reviewing the alphabetical index of the CPT coding manual
    c. Determining which procedures the anesthesiologist performed
    d. Coding from the ICD coding manual

13. [LO 16.1] Which of the following codes would the coder report when a provider performs a surgical procedure that requires anesthesia?
    a. An anesthesia code and a procedure code
    b. A diagnostic code and a procedure code and modifiers
    c. A procedure code with modifiers
    d. An anesthesia code, a procedure code, and any applicable modifiers

14. [LO 16.1] Which of the following are supplementary codes that identify reasons for a patient's encounter other than for a medical illness or injury?
    a. E-codes
    b. Category III codes
    c. V-codes
    d. Physical status modifiers

15. [LO 16.1] Which of the following is the correct way to look up a diagnostic code in the ICD-9-CM coding manual?
    a. First look up the code in the Volume I tabular list for greatest specificity.
    b. First look up the code in the alphabetic index by main term or condition.
    c. Second look up the code in the tabular list in order to code to the greatest degree of specificity.
    d. Both (b) and (c).

16. [LO 16.1] The code(s) _____ describe a patient who has systemic lupus erythematosus with encephalitis.
    a. 710.0
    b. 710.0 and 323.81
    c. 323.81 and 710.0
    d. 323.81

17. [LO 16.1] The code _____ is reported for a patient with acute hemorrhagic pancreatitis.
    a. 577.0
    b. 577.1
    c. 577.2
    d. 095.8

18. [LO 16.1] The code _____ describes uncontrolled diabetes insipidus.
    a. 250.50
    b. 250.00
    c. 253.53
    d. 253.52

**19.** [LO 16.1] The code _____ reports the closure of an intestinal cutaneous fistula.

   **a.** 44602

   **b.** 44640

   **c.** 44700

   **d.** 44227

**20.** [LO 16.1] A physician suspects that her patient has diabetes mellitus. To confirm this she orders a glycosylated hemoglobin test (hemoglobin A1c). What is the correct code for this laboratory test?

   **a.** 83021

   **b.** 83037

   **c.** 83036

   **d.** 83528

**21.** [LO 16.1] The code _____ is used to report chronic adrenal gland insufficiency.

   **a.** 255.41

   **b.** 396.3

   **c.** 428.0

   **d.** 255.5

**22.** [LO 16.1] The code _____ describes an acid perfusion (Bernstein) test performed on a patient with esophagitis.

   **a.** 91020

   **b.** 530.10

   **c.** 530.13

   **d.** 91030

**23.** [LO 16.1] Which of the following codes documents that a patient has participated in smoking cessation classes?

   **a.** 4000F

   **b.** Category I code

   **c.** ICD-9 code

   **d.** 4001F

**24.** [LO 16.1] Which code(s) report a breath test for heart transplantation rejection?

   **a.** Category III code

   **b.** Category II code

   **c.** 0085T

   **d.** Both (*a*) and (*c*)

**25.** [LO 16.1] Procedure code _____ is used to report a routine electroencephalography (EEG) for greater than one hour for a patient with epilepsy.

   **a.** 95812

   **b.** 95827

   **c.** 95813

   **d.** 95950

**26.** [LO 16.1] Procedure code _____ is used to report a 35-year-old patient with end-stage renal disease (ESRD) who receives home dialysis for one month.

   **a.** 90970

   **b.** 90937

   **c.** 90966

   **d.** 90993

**27.** [LO 16.1] Diagnostic code _____ is used to describe a patient who has had a Kaposi varicelliform eruption?

   **a.** 757.33

   **b.** 176.9

   **c.** 054.0

   **d.** 999.0

**28.** [LO 16.1] Which of the following are the correct procedural and diagnostic codes to report for a patient with arachnoiditis requiring a myelography of the brain?

    **a.** 70010 and 322.9

    **b.** 70011 and 036.0

    **c.** 72255 and 322.9

    **d.** 67346 and 094.2

**29.** [LO 16.1] Which of the following are the correct codes to report a mastectomy for a patient with gynecomastia, including the procedure, diagnosis, and anesthesia codes?

    **a.** 00400, 19300, and 611.1

    **b.** 00400, 19303, and 611.1

    **c.** 00402, 19306, and 611.1

    **d.** 00404, 19380, and 611.1

**30.** [LO 16.1] A patient has acute gastritis with nausea and vomiting. Diagnosis codes _____ would be reported to describe this condition.

    **a.** 535.0, 787.02, and 787.03

    **b.** 535.00 and 787.01

    **c.** 535.0 and 787.01

    **d.** 535.00, 787.02, and 787.03

## Applying Your Skills

Assign the code or modifier that best describes each of the following scenarios.

**1.** [LO 16.1] A certified registered nurse anesthetist (CRNA) provides services without medical direction by a physician. Which modifier is added to the codes describing those services? _____

**2.** [LO 16.1] Local anesthesia is originally administered until a complication occurred requiring general anesthesia. Which modifier is added to indicate that while anesthesia is not usually required for a procedure, in a particular case it was necessary? _____

**3.** [LO 16.1] A patient undergoes a full thickness excision of a rectal tumor using transanal endoscopic microsurgery (TEMS). Which code reports the procedure? What type of code is it? _____

**4.** [LO 16.1] A patient's history of coronary artery disease (CAD), with angina symptoms and level of activity, is documented in the medical record. Which code is used to report this? What type of code is it? _____

**5.** [LO 16.1] A patient develops mediastinitis after cardiac surgery, which requires debridement. List the procedure codes to describe the procedure and anesthesia. _____

**6.** [LO 16.1] A physician inserts a dual-lead pacemaker using fluoroscopy. The same physician performs the radiological supervision and interpretation services associated with the pacemaker insertion. Which code(s) describe these services? _____

**7.** [LO 16.1] A patient has a herniated lumbar disk requiring chemonucleolysis under anesthesia. Which code(s) would be used to report this procedure? _____

**8.** [LO 16.1] A diabetic patient with an infected leg abscess requires drug administration by home infusion. Each infusion lasts 1–1½ hours. Which code(s) would be used to describe the service? _____

**9.** [LO 16.1] Which modifier is used to identify a laboratory test performed to identify whether a patient has a genetic abnormality causing Huntington disease, a neurologic, nonneoplastic disease? Where is this modifier found? _____

**10.** [LO 16.1] Which modifier indicates that a clinical diagnostic laboratory test is repeated on the same day to obtain subsequent report test value(s)? _____

**11.** [LO 16.1] A physician performs an incision and drainage procedure on a patient in his office. During the same visit, the physician also performs evaluation and management services for reasons other than the minor surgical procedure performed that day. Which modifier indicates that the E/M procedure is a significant, separately identifiable service performed by the same provider on the same day as a surgical procedure? _____

**12.** [LO 16.1]  A certified registered nurse anesthetist (CRNA) works under the direction of an anesthesiologist. Identify all the appropriate modifier codes that might be necessary to report her service. _____

**13.** [LO 16.1]  A patient with spinal degenerative disk disease undergoes nerve conduction studies to determine which nerves are affected. The coder must identify the nerves tested with specific modifiers. Where would these modifiers be found? _____

**14.** [LO 16.1]  A patient has onychomycosis (nail fungus) of the left thumb and undergoes an avulsion of the nail to treat the infection. Assign the appropriate procedural code and modifier in addition to the diagnostic code to report this condition. _____

**15.** [LO 16.1]  A patient is seen in her physician's office for gastritis, nausea, vomiting, diarrhea, and dehydration. The physician treats the dehydration with an IV infusion lasting 45 minutes. Which code best describes this infusion? _____

# Case Studies

For each of the following scenarios, assign the correct codes and modifiers according to the instructions given in the scenario.

**1.** [LO 16.1]  A patient with a cardiac arrhythmia requires intracardiac catheter ablation to restore normal electrical pathways. A catheter is inserted into the femoral vein and advanced into the heart under fluoroscopic guidance. The catheter is attached to a recording device, an arrhythmia is induced, and the catheter is used to ablate or destroy the abnormal electrical pathway. Once the procedure is completed, a posttest is performed with an attempt to induce an arrhythmia to verify that the procedure was a success. An anesthesiologist provided services throughout the procedure. Report CPT codes for the comprehensive electrophysiological evaluation, mapping the ablation, the ablation itself, and the anesthesia service administered. Report diagnostic codes for these procedures to show proper code linkage for reimbursement.

_____

**2.** [LO 16.1]  A patient with a gunshot wound to the head is admitted to the intensive care trauma unit. He has been declared brain dead. Several of his vital organs will be harvested for donor transplantation, including his kidneys, which will be transplanted into patients with end-stage renal disease. Report the codes and any necessary modifiers to describe the surgery and anesthesia for the donor kidney procedures.

_____

**3.** [LO 16.1]  A 35-year-old female patient with severe right upper quadrant pain arrives in the emergency room. The workup reveals that the patient has a hepatocellular adenoma causing an acute liver hemorrhage. The liver hemorrhage is an acute surgical emergency with the possibility of high mortality. An interventional radiologist performs a transcatheter arterial embolization (TAE) to interrupt the blood supply to the portion of the liver that is hemorrhaging. Identify the codes to report the transcatheter arterial embolization, the anesthesia administration for the procedure, and the diagnostic code for the liver hemorrhage. Be sure to include any add-on codes or modifiers as applicable.

_____

**4.** [LO 16.1]  A routine abdominal ultrasound is performed on a pregnant patient to assess fetal status, including a detailed fetal anatomical examination. It is discovered that the fetus has a large omphalocele that will need to be repaired shortly after birth. Report the diagnosis code that identifies this abnormality, the routine abdominal ultrasound, and the omphalocele repair under general anesthesia. Be sure to include any necessary anesthesia modifiers or qualifying circumstances.

_____

**5.** [LO 16.1] A 66-year-old woman is seen for complaints of headaches and blurred vision. The patient is assessed and a health history is obtained. On physical examination, the patient's blood pressure is 165/95. The physician advises the patient regarding dietary and lifestyle changes and prescribes beta-blockers to control the blood pressure. The physician records these findings and treatment plan in the medical records. The physician reports tracking codes that are used as performance measures of the care provided. What performance measures might be appropriate to report in this situation?

**6.** [LO 16.1] A physician performs high-energy extracorporeal shock wave therapy on a patient's lateral humeral epicondyle under general anesthesia on a patient with lateral epicondylitis of the elbow. List the appropriate diagnosis code, CPT code, and anesthesia code for this procedure. What is the significance of the placement of the CPT code describing the procedure?

**7.** [LO 16.1] A coder is reviewing a patient's medical record in the internal medicine office where she works to determine whether or not it is appropriate to report add-on code 99354 for prolonged physician services. The medical record indicates that the patient presented with an acute condition with moderate distress. The physician performed an initial evaluation, documented the signs and symptoms, and initiated treatment. The physician had intermittent face-to-face contact with the patient over a period of 2 hours. After reviewing the medical records, the coder reviews the CPT manual for guidance on determining whether the prolonged service code is appropriate. Name two locations within the CPT manual that may contain information the coder might find useful. Identify the appropriate CPT index that will aid the coder in making a determination as to whether or not this may or may not be the correct code to use based on the information provided.

**8.** [LO 16.1] A patient with episodic reactive airway disease has been developing full-blown asthma attacks. The patient experiences shortness of breath, chest tightness, and coughing due to airway constriction. In order to effectively treat and prevent further asthma attacks, the physician directs the patient to use a small filtered pneumatic nebulizer. This device requires the use of an administration during treatment. Identify the correct supply code for the administration set used with a small-volume pneumatic nebulizer.

## Thinking It Through

Using your critical-thinking skills, answer the following questions.

**1.** [LO 16.1] Most coders develop their own individual methods to identify all appropriate codes to report the procedures and services described in medical records. There is no single correct method to identify those codes, but the coder should follow a process that identifies all possible code types (CPT, HCPCS, and ICD-9-CM) and applicable modifiers. These methods may change over time. In the space below, describe your current approach to identify the codes to describe procedures and services provided to patients in a healthcare setting.

**2.** [LO 16.1] Describe the major reasons for converting from ICD-9-CM to ICD-10-CM. Identify information that is not available with ICD-9-CM codes but is available with ICD-10-CM codes.

**3.** [LO 16.1] A surgeon scheduled a diagnostic exploratory laparoscopy for a patient with severe abdominal pain. During the procedure he identified the abnormality causing the pain and performed a therapeutic/surgical laparoscopy. Explain in your own words how you would code these two procedures and why you would code it that way. Then identify at least two other types of procedures that follow this same coding convention.

_____

_____

_____

_____

**4.** [LO 16.1] Given what you now know about medical coding and the healthcare field overall, identify some of the biggest challenges to healthcare coding over the next several years.

_____

_____

_____

_____

## Chapter Opening photos:

1: © Patrick Lane/Blend Images/Getty RF; 2: © Fuse/Getty RF; 3: © Peter Dazeley/The Image Bank/Getty; 4: © PhotoAlto/Ale Ventura/Getty RF; 5: © Ken Whitmore/Stone/Getty; 6: © Daniel Allan/Photographer's Choice/Getty RF; 7: © Dana Neely/The Image Bank/Getty; 8: © Jose Luis Pelaez Inc/Blend Images/Getty RF; 9: © Chris Ryan/OJO Images/Getty RF; 10: © Fuse/Getty RF; 11: © Greg Pease/The Image Bank/Getty; 12.1: © MedicImage/Universal Images Group/Collection Mix: Subjects/Getty; 12.2: © Carol & Mike Werner/Visuals Unlimited; 12.3: © Kurt Drubbel/The Agency Collection/Getty RF; 12.4: © Artpartner-Images/Photographer's Choice/Getty; 12.5: © Stockbyte/Getty RF; 12.6: © CMSP/Custom Medical Stock Photo/Getty; 13: © Justin Gollmer/Brand X Pictures/Getty RF; 14: © Ingram Publishing RF; 15: © Chris Ryan/Getty RF; 16 © Janis Christie/Digital Vision/Getty Images/RF